# WATER CODES

# WATER CODES

The Science of Health, Consciousness, and Enlightenment

## Carly Nuday, PhD

Water Ink

California

# CONTENTS

*Life is Water, dancing to the tune of molecules.*
~DR. ALBERT SZENT-GYORGI
NOBEL PRIZE, PHYSIOLOGY OR
MEDICINE

*Ultimately, a theory that would adequately explain the
existence of structured water would also explain the connection
between mind and matter....*
~DR. MARCEL VOGEL
IBM SCIENTIST

# ACKNOWLEDGEMENTS

My life has been a passion of learning and spiritual growth, a continuous evolution and expansion of my mind and spirit. I am so blessed to have been touched by so many throughout my life, guided and supported through the knowledge and insight provided from all types of sources, and the decades of previous research and development from incredible minds. Their work has provided the platform with which we are able to launch into new areas of discovery and application, and were it not for their incredible contributions our society would be severely crippled and we would surely die from lack of knowledge. And so, on the shoulders of giants, I extend my deepest and most humble gratitude to all of these great geniuses, many of who are no longer here to see the culmination of their works.

For Dr. Marcel Vogel, who is the true pioneer of structured water and the greatest crystallographer the world has ever known. Dr. Vogel spent nearly 30 years at IBM developing technology for society, and well recognized the effects crystals and magnets have on energy. After retiring, he dedicated the rest of his days to studying crystals, water, consciousness, and healing.

With great thanks towards the late Joe Blankenship, who provided his amazing encyclopedic knowledge of study and research from so many individuals he encountered throughout his lifetime. An incredible scientist, pioneer, and public health advocate, Joe also helped to keep Marcel and many others' work alive in order to create the field of knowledge we have today.

For the friends and family who have supported and aided me through this incredible journey, you have my eternal love and thanks. This has been an amazing experience, and I am so grateful to have shared it with you.

# SPECIAL NOTICE TO THE READER

I am both at once a scientist and a spiritual theologian, and thus this book reflects both of these traditions by exploring both the science and the spirituality of Water. It examines years of collected information combined with original ideas, and presents a holistic view on the most important fundamentals of Water and its real cycle. By exploring the underlying science and spirituality of Water, expressed in our most sacred texts and demonstrated in our most honest science, we discover that Water is in fact the driving force behind the Laws of Attraction and the Biology of Belief, the Mind-Body-Spirit Connection, and the Storehouse and Mechanism of Consciousness.

While each chapter is worthy of its own book, the information here is compiled in the most brief and simplistic way in order for us to journey through each field and come to the larger picture of how water truly operates, and what this means for our understanding of consciousness and the mind-body-spirit connection. The book begins by covering the basic scientific principles behind structured water, then moves further into the spiritual implications and applications of such knowledge. Enjoy your journey into this fascinating world!

# INTRODUCTION

*Science without Spirituality is lame.*
~EINSTEIN

Water is an amazing substance, the most abundant and yet the most mysterious. It is not only responsible for Life; it is also the key to true health and healing, and the manifesting generator governing the phenomena of the Laws of Attraction and the biology of belief. Within this seemingly simple liquid, we find the first and most powerful computer and fractal antenna, the network in the mind-body-spirit connection, and the storehouse of memory and Consciousness – uncovering both the knowledge of our ancestors and the truth of our existence, all within the realm of Water.

It operates through complex rules of sacred geometry (or shapes), the movement and conduction of energy and information transfer and storage, and although it is one of the longest and most studied substances on our planet, most people – including the scientists who study it – know little to nothing about it. In fact, you will be hard-pressed to find anyone who can tell you Water is the mechanism of action for the *Secret* and the *Law of Attraction*, or that Water is a fractal antenna computing energy and consciousness to manifest and determine the expression of your DNA. You will be even harder pressed to find anyone to explain *how* Water is responsible for such amazing phenomena that is so central to our existence. These are essential truths that you will find within these pages, with implications that touch the deepest parts of our bodies, minds, and spirits.

So vital is Water to Life, there is not a culture that has existed which has not had an intimate relationship with it, recognizing Water as the most critical ingredient in their survival and prosperity. And yet the true nature of Water, the true facts behind its properties as a substance, its relationship to consciousness, and its methods of action in the body, have often been ignored, overlooked, or even denied. The true abilities of Water and its real connection to our health have been so disregarded, in fact, that it makes one wonder whether such incredible information is being purposely obscured from the public realm of insight. After years of investigation, research, and development, this author has concluded that such blatant denial, career persecution, and information withholding must have likely been intentional.

When one truly recognizes the role of Water in health, healing, and consciousness, one begins to understand their body and their environment in new ways; ways that allow us to see the true source of symptoms, and treat preventatively for the first time, giving the power of health back to the individual. It allows us to see our consciousness, and for the first time truly understand the impacts thought and actions have on our bodies, minds, and spirits. Seeing the relationship between energy, our Water, and our health, allows us to step into that feedback loop in a proactive way. With this information, we are no longer victims of the energetic processing of our Water cycle. Instead, we are able to find and take our place as Co-Creators, participating in the creation of our health and longevity and experiencing the expansion of our consciousness and spirit.

# PART I

# THE UNTOLD MYSTERY OF WATER

# CHAPTER 1

# THE UNTOLD MYSTERY OF WATER

---

*Water is the driving force of All of Nature.*
~LEONARDO DA VINCI

Water is the essence of Life, the most fundamental substance to our existence. Once thought to be unique to our planet and now recognized as quite pervasive throughout the Universe, Water is far more than the simple aqueous substance we are taught in academia. It has incredible, unexpected, and anomalous properties, which chemistry and physics say it should not have. In fact, the laws of both chemistry and physics predict that water would not even be present on Earth in liquid form, and yet without it Life would not exist. It has been studied since study began, and worshipped by countless tribes and cultures. It is the magic behind the Fountain of Youth, the great Waters of the Lourdes, and the spirit of baptism. Its movement drove the mechanics of the actions of the pyramids, and has determined the success or failure of villages and cities throughout time. It is central to nearly every religious ritual and ceremony; considered by our most sacred texts, revered saints, honored prophets, and wisest sages to be the source of spiritual life, physical health, and the very foundation of our Universe. Water, older than life itself, is honored and discussed in every Creation story ever told. Still we are captivated by its amazing mystery and power, revering this substance throughout history, *without even understanding what Water is* – even though it is the primary substance of which we are made – *99% by molecular count.*

> *We know almost nothing about Water.*
> ~DR. VLADIMIR VOEIKOV
> BIOPHYSICIST
> MOSCOW UNIVERSITY

The truth about Water is astounding. What it reveals about life, consciousness, and energy is remarkable. We find ourselves at a time when technology allows us to see more than we ever thought possible, as in the advancements of MRI and NRI (Magnetic or Nuclear Resonance Imaging) technology which reveal reactions, expressions, and computations among water molecules in response to energy and consciousness. Water molecules are *incredibly* small, yet today's technologies make it possible to physically view the structure and shape they make as they arrange themselves, allowing us to compare the shape and structure of the water molecules inside of the cells, the bloodstream, and even those surrounding the DNA strands. We are able to compare water from different sources, different cells, and different people, viewing the differences in molecular arrangement and properties, which reveal astounding relationships between the patterns of the water molecules and their sources. Water from diseased cells looks different than water from healthy cells, just as water from sacred sites forms different patterns in their molecules than water from your tap. Never before have we had the technology available to actually view the molecular structure and correlate it with the water's properties. Never before have we been able to collect and compare water samples from so many different sources in the world, and never before has science allowed such insight into the deeper spirituality discussed by our ancestors.

Science is the spirituality of "rational" and Western thought. Traditionally, it has existed as a model to reduce the phenomena of our Universe into logical and consistent rules and laws. Yet as the scientific and technological breakthroughs continue to occur at exploding exponential rates, the lines between science and spirituality begin to blur. Quantum mechanics teaches us that if even one thing was random, the entire Universe would fall apart, lending much support to the Divine Plan of most spiritual and religious traditions. Beliefs of multiple religious systems find scientific advancements confirming their ancient traditions. Through the avenue of Science, many are finding their way to Spirit, with an understanding and appreciation for the magical mystery of consciousness and existence. And yet still many are lost or confused, finding contradictions they are unable to overcome without a greater knowledge of the Science of Spirituality, and the Spirituality of Science.

There exists, through acknowledging the gifts of both scientific and spiritual traditions, and marrying their deepest and truest fundamentals, a bridge that unifies these two apparently warring groups. Through this union, we find a synergy of information, where the resulting understanding is much greater than the sum of its parts. We find the physics behind the laws of manifestation through the consciousness and computing power of Water, the structures and patterns of consciousness that determine laws of attraction and magnetism, and the explainable models of the energetic fields of our environments. We recognize the true messages of our ancient texts and teachings, profound spiritual science and universal truth hidden in the depths of unrealized metaphor, their full meanings revealed only when viewed through the lens of knowledge. This is a path of exploration, of expanded perceptions, and of exponential growth and development. Through this path, we understand the real hidden messages in Water, and discover the true secrets within the Water Codes.

# CHAPTER 2

# LESSONS FROM ACADEMIA

---

Taught in school, we examined a glass of 'simple water' and learned that it is the only substance to exists as a solid, a liquid, and a gas in natural form, and is an arrangement of two hydrogen atoms and one oxygen atom. Moving further into chemistry, we learned that these atoms are held together to form this liquid/solid/gaseous substance via covalent hydrogen bonding, and that it made a great medium and solvent. And that was that. But what if it is not so simple? Most have never even *heard* of other forms of 'water', for example $H_3O$ or $H_3O_2$, or water's *van der Waals bonds*, the term used to describe the attraction between water molecules caused by electrostatic force (i.e. the forces between atoms and particles that are caused by their electrical charges).

Instead, Water's most intriguing anomalous properties were likely ignored, as science is unable to explain why water has the highest surface tension of any liquid, is the greatest solvent on earth, and defies gravity every time it rises through the trunks of trees. Perhaps Water's great uniqueness was hinted at in the classic verbatim that water, like energy, cannot be created or destroyed, and that the water we have here today on earth is the same amount, atom for atom, which has always been here

– both theories highly controversial, but taught, at least to me and others I know, at a young age. But Water's great collection of anomalous properties – over 60 unexplainable properties according to modern chemistry and physics – has been often ignored and untaught. The unexplainable properties of water, the most pervasive substance on our planet, fly in the face of modern physics and call into question the very 'Laws' on which our entire scientific system is based. When the Laws of Physics fail miserably to apply to the most common substance on our planet, one must question their legitimacy and recognize that the rules of physics do not operate as we once believed. While one would think that science would be forever embracing new ideas and discovery, it is an incredibly difficult task to undo the branches of sciences from the fundamentals on which they are based, no matter *how* wrong they are, and we are perhaps not as far from the days of Galileo as we would like to believe. Career persecution is rampant in the fields of discovery, and thus a great deal of gathered knowledge and research on the many properties of water also go ignored, not yet acknowledged by mainstream science.

> *Water is the most studied material on Earth but it is remarkable to find that the science behind its behavior and function are so poorly understood (or even ignored), not only by people in general, but also by scientists working with it everyday. The small size of its molecule belies the complexity of its actions and its singular capabilities. Liquid water's unique properties and chameleonic nature seem to fit ideally into the requirements for life as can no other molecule.*
> ~MARTIN CHAPLIN
> PROFESSOR OF APPLIED SCIENCE

LONDON SOUTH BANK UNIVERSITY

Even the most basic properties of water don't conform to the rules of physics. If water contracted rather than expanding when freezing, as most compounds do, it would sink and destroy life. Instead, water contracts at 3.9°C, an anomaly that causes the spring and fall turnover of lakes in temperate climates. Lake turnover occurs when the deeper waters are exchanged with surface waters, a natural yearly cycling of nutrients and oxygen that are so critical for lake life. Without this anomalous property (called "anomalous" because it is unexpected), lake life would not even exist, nor would the plethora of diverse forms of life within its ecosystem and all of the ecosystems around it that are dependent upon its water system. The only lakes to exist would be in the tropic zones, where seasonal turnover occurs through violent tropical storms.

The rules of physics also expect the boiling temperature of water to be -70°C, (rather than 100°C, depending on the conditions) and that it should freeze around -100°C instead of 0°C – again, depending on the conditions, as water has been shown to have no static or set boiling and freezing point. Yet the structural bonding in water allows it to exist outside of the gaseous state the rules of chemistry and physics expect it to be in, and thankfully so, or there would be no liquid water on Earth at our temperatures. And these are just some of the growing number of Water's anomalous properties.

To be frank, with all the credit and discovery attributed to the broad field of Science, one would assume that after all this time the schools of the sciences would have a well founded definition of what Water even *is*. But no such definition has been able to include and account for the amazing properties of water, and the answers postulated by science are incomplete, typically explaining away some anomalies while being in direct opposition to other properties. Why, for example, is water heaviest at 4°C, and what makes it freeze at 0°C? Why does it sometimes *not* freeze at 0°C? Why is some water "lighter" than other water? Why does "super-cooled" water have different properties than "regular" water?

More importantly, perhaps, to the general population and reaching further than mainstream science is comfortable going, what makes some water so much different than other water? Why does some water, whether homeopathic, treated with a form of subtle energy (that energy which is unseen, and yet we witness its effects and thus know it exists) or magnetism, sourced from a sacred site (i.e. Lourdes, France), or otherwise 'differentiated' water, have documented healing effects, and exhibit different properties all together from 'other' water?

These water sources have been demonstrated to produce different ice crystal growth, affect the growth of other crystalline substances, change the color of specific colloid minerals, absorb different spectra of light, be measurably lighter than other water, and exhibit a variety of other changes in properties. They also come with thousands of years of anecdotal evidence of miraculous healings, and even well documented studies in modern eras.

Upon investigation, one learns there seem to be two different *types* of water – 'structured', 'ordered', or 'organized' water, which intelligently arranges its molecules in crystalline patterns, and 'un-structured' or 'bulk' water, which has dis-ordered molecules – and these waters exist in their various degrees. These two different types of water exhibit different enough characteristics to nearly be considered two completely different substances, except that they still remain comprised of the compound we know as $H_2O$. Un-structured water, also known as 'bulk', 'un-organized', or 'dead' water, appears to be more like the simple glass of liquid we are taught in school, whereas structured water, also known as 'hexagonal', 'organized', 'living', 'sacred', 'holy', or 'healing' water, appears to be a much more mysterious substance, even though it comprises the most of our biology. It behaves much more unusually than its less-ordered counterpart 'bulk' water, it exhibits more anomalous properties the more ordered and structured it becomes, and it is much more critical to *all* of Life's many processes.[1]

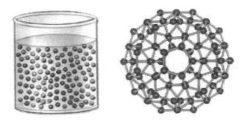

Fig. 1: Random molecules in a glass (left) vs.
Organized water molecule cluster (right).
*Cluster image: Martin Chaplin, London South Bank University*

It is this aspect of water, its structuring capabilities,

---

1. Errington, JR, Debenedetti, PG. Relationship Between Structural Order and the Anomalies of Liquid Water." *Nature.* Jan 18;409 (6818):318-21. Department of Chemical Engineering, Princeton University, 2001.

which gives rise to its remarkable features – from its ability to defy physics, to its ability to store information, memory, and cause healing – and it's this aspect that is getting so much attention in the marketplace. There are a growing number of products being sold today to ionize, alkalize, magnetize, intentionalize, and vortex water to improve its pH and absorption, hydration potential and 'molecular cluster formation', energy charge density, and *structure*, in order to improve its ability to penetrate cells and amplify effects in the body – i.e. water's 'bio-availability and function'. But for all the language and research discussed by such marketers (some more true than others), there is still an inadequate understanding or knowledge of *what* structured water really is, really does, or really can do.

It is imperative, if we are to understand our bodies, our health, and our life, our consciousness, energy, and Universe, that we expand our understanding of Water. This requires a holistic view, combining science and spirituality, bridging cultural and ancient knowledge with the advancements of today. Perhaps if science were to look at the properties of water and its behavior in the context of the historical knowledge left by our ancestors, their definition of water could begin to look more complete and the possibilities of its application expansive and near limitless.

Like so many other great discoveries we've made about our Universe and experience – from the order of our solar system, which is accurately depicted in several ancient traditions, to the effect of positive thinking on health, a topic discussed for centuries in sacred texts and scriptures – we find evidence of ancient knowledge surrounding water's amazing properties in cultures throughout time and space on Earth. It is the incredible nature of *structured water* that holds the meaning and the power behind holy or sacred water sites and rituals of blessings and cleansings. In *structured water,* we find the mechanisms and the abilities the ancients recognized and revered in water, and through understanding water in its *true form and function,* we begin to develop different and deeper meaning and relations to the religious and sacred literature referencing its characteristics, abilities, and use.

This book aims to answer the question of what structured water *really is* in a clear way, by providing evidence and research of aqueous knowledge and discovery throughout history, shining light on the remarkable qualities and responsiveness of Water, and put it together in context to show how Water works as *energy,* as an *interface,* as a *fractal antenna of information,* and as the *storehouse of consciousness.* Having understood the *science* behind structured water, it then aims to shed light on what our ancestors were *really* saying about water, through both their texts and traditions, now having the scientific language to understand how these processes are capable. Only then can we begin to understand how Water holds the greatest value for health, wellness, and longevity, and what the science of Structured Water can tell us about the energetics of our Universe. As we grow this understanding, we begin to see that water's anomalous properties are perhaps not so anomalous, and we open ourselves up to explore how the mechanics of Water allow us to examine the fundamental Laws of Energy and Consciousness in our Universe, the Laws on which our existence is based.

CHAPTER 3

# THE SURPRISING SCIENTIFIC HISTORY

*Anyone who can solve the problems of water will be worthy of two Nobel Prizes: one for Peace, and one for Science.*
~JOHN F. KENNEDY

In the mainstream public, there seems to be three schools of thought regarding water's structuring capacities. One group accepts the explanations given by documentaries such as *Water, the Great Mystery*, the works of Masaru Emoto, or the marketers of structured water products. Another group echoes the sentiments of snow crystal author Kenneth Libbrecht of Caltech University, who essentially says, "don't be ridiculous, it's just water". The third group has no idea all together, and has likely never even heard of 'structured water' before. But this is amongst the mainstream public, whose opinions and ideas are often pre-determined by media influence and exposure. What about the scientists?

The relationship between scientists and structured water goes back much further than any mainstream public exposure. In fact, the Structure of Water has a long history with the Nobel Prize, prestigious scientific journals, and documented, credible research, making one wonder how so many can be critical of its discussion. Three Nobel Prizes were awarded in the 1990's for work relating to 'clustered', 'organized', or 'structured' water, namely involving DNA, intracellular fluids, cellular communication, and protein folding. They discovered that healthy DNA is surrounded by water in a crystalline matrix (i.e. *structured water*), an incredible finding that will be expanded upon in later chapters.[1] Notice that these discoveries related to structured water have to do with the critical functions of structured water within living organisms – from cellular communication to DNA integrity. As it turns out, Nobel Prize Laureates have known for quite some time that the structure of our *bio-water* – the water within our bodies – is highly organized and crystalline in nature, and that *this intelligent organization is critical to every single bio-chemical-electro reaction in the body.* This is in no way any form of pseudo-science, rather it is science at its finest.

Dr. Albert Szent-Gyorgyi, who won the Nobel Prize in 1937 for vitamin C and is held as the father of bio-chemistry, long recognized the importance of the structure of the water within our cells. He scoffed at mainstream science's ignorance of this fact, stating,

*Biology has forgotten the intracellular water, or it did not discover it, as yet.*

Dr. Szent-Gyorgyi went further, acknowledging the critical role of structured cellular waters and our development of understanding:

1. Dr. Mu Shik Jhon. *The Water Puzzle and the Hexagonal Key: Scientific Evidence of Hexagonal Water and Its Positive Influence on Health.* Utah: Uplifting Press Inc., 2004.

*Since the structure of Water is the essence of all Life, the man who can control that structure in cellular systems will change the world.*

This statement by Dr. Szent-Gyorgyi was decades ahead of other scientists, and is still ahead of many today. It was not, however, ahead of one of his peers, whose work likely influenced Dr. Szent-Gyorgyi's. Fellow Nobel Prize winner Linus Pauling remains the only man to receive two unshared Nobel Prizes, and one of the only two people in the world to receive two shared Nobel Prizes. In 1935, Pauling presented his theories on *water's memory*, one of its most amazing properties wherein water *rearranges its structure of molecular arrangement in order to encode, transmit, and integrate new information, akin to storing 'memory'.* His concepts behind anesthesia and the water molecules in the brain are only just now becoming celebrated by neuroscientists, who finally have access to technology which supports his understanding.[2] He postulated his theory on water's structure long before it was demonstrated by Jacques Benveniste (and more recently by a group of French physicists), whose research in the late 1980's on structured water led to the conclusion that *the configuration of molecules in water was biologically active.* In demonstrating that the arrangement of molecules of water was "biologically active," what Jacque Benveniste was *really* saying was that the structure of water *had an affect on living organisms.* These findings lent support to the tradition of homeopathy – a method of natural healing which uses incredibly diluted solutions of organic materials such as plants, diluted to the point

2. Nakada, Tsutomu. Neuroscience of Water Molecules: A Salute to Professor Linus Carl Pauling. *Journal of Cytotechnology*. April 2009; 59(3): 145-152.

where only water remains and none of the original matter. This 'water' dilution is then used as the remedy. Because all we can detect in the substance is water, up to this point there was no scientific support that one remedy was any different from another remedy – and yet, if a person had malaria and took the homeopathic remedy for scarlet fever, it would do nothing, however if the person took the homeopathic remedy proper for their condition (in this case for malaria), they would be cured. How could this be? Both substances were assumed to be simple water, and having no particle matter of the plant itself – not even a single atom – there is nothing that would suggest the remedies were any different from each other, other than the impressive anecdotal evidence for homeopathy. The reason the substances are different is because they carry different structural patterns and arrangements in their water molecules, which has a profound impact on health. This is what Benveniste was referring to when he discussed the configuration, or shape, of water molecules as being *biologically active,* i.e. having an effect on living organisms. Unfortunately, Benveniste, like many others, was highly persecuted by the professional community for such 'fringe' notions, and his publications were removed from the prestigious scientific journal *Nature* in which they had been published. Still, experiments demonstrating water's memory have continued, as have the search for the answers as to why water exhibits this ability, what applications this knowledge can have, and what larger implications this may present for our understanding of ourselves, our lives, our environments, and our Universe.

Nearly all of the scientific discovery and contributions regarding structured water have stayed under the public's radar and out of the mainstream media and the realm of general information. It has also, for the most part, stayed very 'chemical-physical', discussing the *properties* of structured water while largely staying out of the realm of memory, consciousness, or homeopathy. Theories about how water is able to express so many unexpected and anomalous properties are still being formulated, and it was not until 2001 that an article was published in the prestigious scientific journal *Nature* which successfully demonstrated (through computer simulation) that water's anomalous properties "arise from water's propensity for organization and structure."[3] The work was also featured in the Princeton Weekly Bulletin, and structured water scientists everywhere were likely shaking their heads in amazement at the elementary level at which so many scientists continue to operate. This is certainly important research, exampled by the article's implication of the many potentials for use in the preservation of pharmaceutical drugs – considering that *organizing and structuring water in a specific fashion alters its properties to such a degree as to promote stable preservation of substances.* What is disappointing though, is that the article quotes a Boston University professor as "an authority on the anomalous properties of water", who states that the researchers "link[ed] ideas that no one had ever dreamed were related."[4] To all structured water scientists, this is insulting, because it implies that the discovery that water's structure is responsible for its anomalous properties is somehow a novel idea. The computer simulation, perhaps, is a novel development, but the links between the recognized and unrecognized anomalous

3. Errington, JR, Debenedetti, PG. 2001.
4. Schultz, Steven. Pouring Over Mystery. *Princeton Weekly Bulletin, Vol. 90, No. 17,* Princeton University Press, February 19, 2001.

properties of water as rising from its propensity for structure and organization have been made for decades.

Meanwhile, other research indicates that the possibilities of structured water appear limitless, as recently demonstrated by Luc Montagnier, a Nobel Prize winning biologist, in a stunning and fascinating experiment. Montagnier successfully conducted an experiment in which DNA appeared to replicate itself between the test tubes, *through the water*. In the experiment, Montagnier and his team took two test tubes, one containing a tiny piece of bacterial DNA and the other containing pure water, and surrounded them with a weak electromagnetic field that is similar to the energy waves naturally emitted by the Earth. The results of their experiment were phenomenal, and speak volumes towards confirming what so many people are already understanding about Water and energy transference, demonstrating long held (and long denied) theories.

While we will explore *electromagnetic fields* and *frequencies* more later on, let us take a moment to more clearly define and understand these terms. These words have made their way out of the scientific arena and are becoming much more common to the general public as people begin to develop and use the language necessary to creatively explore, discuss, and expand our knowledge of these concepts. In essence, everything emits vibrating waves of energy. We refer to these as *electromagnetic fields* or *electromagnetic frequencies*, but they are really just vibrating patterns of energy waves (which are both *electric* and *magnetic* in nature – hence the term 'electro-magnetic'). All perceivable energies in the Universe are considered electro-magnetic energies, and this relationship is inseparable – you cannot generate electricity without also having a corresponding magnetic field, and every magnetic field also carries electric energy.

These vibrating waves of electric and magnetic energy can be measured by how many times the wave pattern repeats itself in a single second, which is called its *Hertz* value. Thus 1 Hertz, or 1Hz, is one cycle of the pattern per second, while 7Hz is seven repetitions of the pattern per second. The electromagnetic field used by Montagnier was 7Hz, which repeats its wave pattern 7 times every second, and is very close to the same 'electromagnetic frequency', or vibrating energy emission, that is generated by Earth's electromagnetic field. The vibrating energies emitted by the Earth's electromagnetic field *reverberate*, or resonate, in the Earth's ionosphere. This means that the energy waves emitted from the Earth echo, in a sense, in the ionosphere around our planet, the way the sound of a church bell resonates in the Cathedral, or the sound of an opera singer reverberates and echoes in a concert hall.

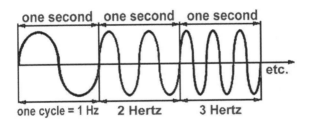

Fig. 2: Hertz (Hz): number of cycles
or repetitions of the pattern, per second

Vibrating energy waves, measured by the *number of repetitions per second of their specific pattern*, are assigned a number on the "electromagnetic scale" according to this pattern. The electromagnetic scale is the ruler of measurement for all types of perceivable energies – which is to say that all perceivable energies are both *electric* and *magnetic* in nature and can thus be assigned a number on the ruler. This number is referred to as its *frequency* – for example, the frequency of your radio station, where 92.5 is a specific electromagnetic wave pattern projected through the air. Visible and non-visible lights are certain frequencies (or vibrating energy wave patterns), as is audible sound for the human ear, or the unique frequency on which your cell phone operates. Observations of the 'frequency', or the vibrating wave pattern, emitted by the Earth's electromagnetic field were first documented by Nikola Tesla in 1899. It was this observation that allowed Tesla to form the basis for his idea of wireless energy transmission (the original Wi-Fi) using the Earth's natural extremely low frequencies. Tesla was successful in utilizing the Earth's naturally resonating energy emissions, and created successful free wireless energy transmission long before today's Wi-Fi, capable of powering all cities and even vehicles with abundant, free, and natural wireless energy transmission, as he demonstrated numerous times – before the American Institute of Electrical Engineers at Columbia College in 1891, again while powering the entire Chicago World's Fair in 1893, and also to the National Electric Light Association that same year.[5] [6] [7] In 1896 he succeeded in wireless transmission over a 48-kilometer distance (about 30 miles).[8]

5. Tesla, Nikola. *Experiments with Alternating Currents of Very High Frequency, and Their Application to Methods of Artificial Illumination.* Delivered before the American Institute of Electrical Engineers, Columbia College, N.Y., May 20, 1891.

6. Barrett , John Patrick. *Electricity at the Columbian Exposition.* Chicago: R.R. Donnelley and Sons Co, 1894. 168-169.

7. *Nikola Tesla, 1856-1943.* IEEE History Center, IEEE, Lecture-demonstration. St Louis, M.O., 1893.

8. Anderson, Leland, ed. *Nikola Tesla on His Work with Alternating Currents and*

The concept of transmitting energy wirelessly using the Earth's naturally occurring vibrating energy emissions or 'wave forms' is significant on its own, even without Tesla's genius of tapping into the energy produced by the lightning in our ionosphere to generate free energy. The wireless energy transmission systems of today use *much* faster energy waves, in the several hundreds of Giga-Hertz (meaning they are *billions* of cycles per second and are in the 'microwave' range – as in microwave cookers) rather than extremely low frequency of the Earth's natural average of 7.83 cycles per second wave emissions, also called the "Schumann Resonance" after the German physicist Winfried Schumann. These 'extremely high frequency' electromagnetic fields, which are increasingly projected into our environments and communities at unprecedented rates, are artificially created and their use is extremely controversial. They have been repeatedly found to be destructive to our health and consciousness, the mechanics of which will be explained in this book, and we are being continually and exponentially exposed to such frequencies without our knowledge or permission. Extremely low frequencies, however, like those of the Earth's natural electromagnetic field vibration, are found to not only be beneficial for life, but also *necessary for its support.* Experiments where plants, animals, and individuals were denied exposure to the Schumann Resonance of Earth's natural electromagnetic field all resulted in a rapid and steady decline in health until they were again exposed to Earth's electromagnetic field. These types of experiments are only possible through space travel, or the construction of rooms and cages created from materials that will block all forms of electromagnetic radiation (even those from the Earth) referred to as *Faraday cages*. It has been argued that the severe deterioration of the health and physical condition experienced by the early astronauts were largely the result of being outside of this resonating field, and that this problem was solved by introducing a *'magnetic pulse generator'* which simulates the Schumann Resonance aboard all space shuttles, emitting energy waves that are similar to those emitted by the Earth. Thus, we see that electromagnetic frequencies can have a *massive* impact on our health and well-being.

Returning to Montagnier's experiment, we find that his use of the same natural energy waves of the Earth was critical to his success. Eighteen hours later, Montagnier's two test tubes, one with the tiny piece of bacterial DNA and the other of the pure water, were examined. What was observed was remarkable, shocking nearly all 'mainstream' scientists while celebrated by nearly all 'fringe' scientists. After eighteen hours of the tubes simply sitting next to each other, with the same type of energy waves emitted by the Earth surrounding it, the DNA was now detectable not only in the original test tube which contained it, *but also in the test tube containing pure water.* The experiment was tested against several other groups with different variables (i.e. type of energy wave, or duration of time), but the only time the DNA was able to imprint into the other test tube of pure water was when exposed to the same energy wave pattern emitted by the Earth for an eighteen-hour time span.

The implications demonstrated by such an experiment are large and numerous. For one, it indicates a *quantum effect* (which simply means an event where particles or atoms do not behave according to Newtonian physics and are not 'obeying the rules'), a necessary cumulative effect of time required for success, and potentially even a type of manifestation or 'teleportation-type' phenomena, where the DNA was able to manifest or imprint a copy of itself into water across space with no apparent 'mode of transportation' or way of getting there without direct interaction. The problems with accepting such implications are fairly obvious. *Quantum phenomena*, studied by scientists in the growing field of quantum physics, are assumed to manifest in imperceivable fractions of a second, i.e. *pico-seconds* (one-trillionth of a second), as opposed to *growing* into manifest over a period of time so extended as eighteen hours. They are also typically observable only at extremely low temperatures approaching absolute zero, whereas Montagnier was conducting his tests in a room temperature environment. Both of these facts are huge contradictions to classical quantum physics theories, and will send them back to the drawing board to revisit some of their primary fundamentals. And because the original DNA sample had to be diluted many times for the experiment to work, it lends great support to the tradition of homeopathy, the specific natural therapy system that was also supported by Benveniste's work. Recall that in homeopathy, a substance is diluted out of a solution into pure water so many times that it becomes *chemically undetectable* and not a single physical atom of the original substance remains. This, then, is the remedy – pure water considered to have been energetically imprinted, or *structured,* with the energetic signature of the original substance. While often ridiculed by Western medicine, which relies on expensive, patentable, and profitable pharmaceutical drugs, homeopathy has a substantial amount of underground support and an impressive history of success. Homeopathy has a longstanding presence in Britain's national health care system, with over 40% of doctors referring patients to homeopathic physicians and the support and use of homeopathy by the British Royal Family since the 1830's. In Europe, homeopathic medicine is so widely practiced by physicians it is no longer appropriate to consider it 'alternative medicine', used regularly by 30% of French doctors and 20% of German doctors, while nearly half of Dutch physicians consider them effective.[9]

In Montagnier's experiment, the DNA was energetically copied into the water much in the way that homeopathic remedies are energetically imprinted – that is to say, they are *structurally encoded into the Water*, the mechanics of which will be discussed in the next chapter as we explore water's propensity to exhibit a *liquid crystal state*. Here, the structure of the water and its arrangement of molecules had been changed, or encoded, with the information of the DNA or the homeopathic remedy. Because the original DNA sample was so highly diluted, it couldn't be chemically detected. Thus, when it came time to examine the test tube of pure water for the presence of DNA, the scientists used a method of adding enzymes to the water in order to see if they would react to the presence of DNA (called a *polymerase chain reaction,* polymerase referring to the type of enzyme used). When the enzymes were added to the test tube of pure water, they reacted as if they were in the presence of DNA, and thus the scientists concluded that the highly diluted DNA was actually present in the water. When one is familiar with the science of structured water, as you will be after reading this book, it is easy to understand that the information of the DNA was encoded into the pattern and the intelligent arrangement of the water molecules

---

9. Thayer, Jeff. *The DNA and Structured Water Interfaces.* 2011.

themselves, and may not have been actually 'present' in protein-form. Because it is the *structure* of a substance that is important in chemical reactions, and not its actual chemical ingredients, the structure of the DNA information in the water was the only thing necessary for the enzymes to initialize a reaction – because the water molecules themselves had become *arranged* and *shaped* with the information of the DNA, which is really all that matters. That it is the *structure* rather than the *chemical ingredients* that determine chemical reactions will be supported and expanded upon in further chapters, here we will simply state the fact.

In the early 1980's, prior to Benveniste and long before any of today's science and remarkable demonstrations of structured water phenomenon, Dr. Marcel Vogel, former IBM researcher and world-renowned crystallographer, was studying the relationship between water and consciousness – particularly the effect of consciousness on the structure of water. While working for IBM for nearly 30 years, Marcel Vogel developed the technology behind today's liquid crystal displays, phosphor-luminescence, and magnetic hard drive encodings, fathering much of today's crystal and computer based technology. He left IBM to further investigate the water and consciousness connection, as well as the connection between consciousness, energy, and living organisms, which led him to collaborate with Cleve Backster in the phenomenal work demonstrating the deeply connected consciousness of plants using lie detectors. Dr. Vogel began successfully using spectrophotometers to measure changes in waters in reaction to thought and intention, demonstrating water's liquid crystal properties in response to consciousness and energy. He continued to further explore the implications and applications of these properties before his death in 1991. Prior to his death, Marcel developed tools with *water resonance* (discussed in later chapters), which allow for greater information transfer to the water and thus to the bodies of individuals for healing. These tools held great potentials for the ability to deliver specific frequencies and information to an individual, and even held potentials as a delivery system for pharmaceutical drug information, which could allow patients to require less or no ingestion of the drug itself while still receiving its therapeutic benefits. Unfortunately, Dr. Vogel had an untimely heart attack just 6 months after discussing these potentials, preventing him from its further development. But the phenomena of water's responsiveness to consciousness finally gained mainstream attention some 13 years later, through the work of Masaru Emoto featured in the hit film, "What the Bleep Do We Know?!", a mainstream documentary discussing consciousness and quantum physics. Dr. Emoto specialized in taking photographs of ice crystals to demonstrate the effects of various stimuli (consciousness, language, intention, music, environment, etc.) on water by flash freezing it into its solid crystalline state in order to view the change in molecular formation after exposure to the stimulus.

In the 1960's, Dr. Bernard Grad at the McGill University in Montreal stumbled upon water's ability to store information and 'charge' while researching psychic phenomena. Grad was more interested in researching whether or not psychic healers were working outside of the realm of placebo effects, rather than studying the water itself, but his studies and findings are quite exemplary of water's ability to change with consciousness and intention. Grad conducted multiple well-designed experiments demonstrating that healers, and also magnetic fields, had positive effects on water as measured through its ability to accelerate plant growth. He also inadvertently demonstrated the *de-structuring* abilities of negative energies on the structure of water's molecular arrangement, by having the water treated intentionally by severely depressed psychiatric patients (as opposed to a healer's intentions) and examining the rate of growth suppression in seedlings. Chemical analysis on the water treated by healers and/or magnets indicated it had been *structured* – infrared spectroscopy revealed the atomic bond angle of the water had shifted and surface tension had been reduced, both indicating structural changes in the molecular formation. Several researchers since, including Douglas Dean and Edward Brame, as well as Stephan Schwartz and others, have replicated Grad's findings of changes in water treated by healers.[10]

Grad's work primarily focused on healers and psychics, rather than exploring or discussing the *method of action* of water's reaction to different consciousness stimuli. Benveniste's work was criticized for the language within its publication that provided support for the fundamental theory behind homeopathy (the description of the water being *biologically active*), but had little to do with the responsiveness of water to consciousness. Dr. Marcel Vogel's work, on the other hand, demonstrated quite clearly and scientifically water's responsiveness to consciousness and intention. Today the work of Dr. Masaru Emoto, as well as other less known researchers provides us with visual representations and aids to support our understanding of the amazing phenomena of water's responsiveness. Emoto's work is mainly criticized for not being 'scientific enough', for not following 'proper

10. Gerber, Richard, M.D. *Vibrational Medicine*. Third Edition. Rochester, Vermont: Bear and Co., 2001.

scientific methods', and for publishing his work privately rather than publically, where it could go under the intense scrutiny – like Benveniste's – desired by the mainstream scientific world. He is also criticized for having been excessively selective about those working on his project, as traditional science says his experiments should be repeatable and not dependent on the individuals conducting the experiment. These criticisms, however, hold little weight when viewed holistically and are truly not well-founded skepticism. Anyone familiar with scientific persecution, such as that experienced by Benveniste and countless others can empathize with Emoto's decision for private publication. More importantly, quantum physics now confirms that the observer directly affects the outcome manifested in reality. Under this model, we have to accept that the individual conducting an experiment has a measurable effect on the result, thus Masaru Emoto has demonstrated an astute understanding of this potential impact. Although formerly not so eloquently put, it appears that Emoto and his team intentionally chose individuals with a high level of consciousness, clarity, and awareness, who demonstrate the ability and propensity to be open-minded and harmonious with their work. This is the best type of approach to observing nature, and every naturalist will affirm this. Unfortunately science, whose entire premise is built on finding the truth through observing nature, operates on principles of a scientific method that is in direct contradiction to this approach. The very basis of predicting an outcome before the event, and then exercising and changing the experiment in order to demonstrate the predicted event, operates directly on observer manifestation where the scientist is blatantly interfering with the result of an experiment with a predetermined conscious perception, creating immediate bias in the action of the experiment. The criticism aimed at Emoto for selecting specific individuals to conduct the research really demonstrates a prevailing ignorance in the scientific community about how the Universe really works, the very thing they are supposed to understand (better than most). And while Emoto has also been criticized for not publishing *all* of the photos taken of specific ice crystals, leading some to theorize that he selectively chose photos that supported his message while omitting ones that didn't, too much similar work has been demonstrated by other researchers. Some, such as Professor Konstantin Korotkov in Russia, has demonstrated remarkably similar photography work, while others like Laurent Costa, of France, has produced photographs of a quite different visual nature than Emoto's. Professor David Schweitzer was likely the first to photograph water's responsiveness to consciousness, and his work pre-dates Emoto's by several years. These men's work and others support Emoto's photographic research with similar observations regarding the structuring or de-structuring effects of different stimuli, particularly that of consciousness, on water.

The photographic work of such researchers is beautiful, and is an invaluable visual aid for viewing the way Water expresses the way it is affected by different types of energy and consciousness, but it does little to explain the true meaning, functions, methods, and implications of this phenomenon. Dr. Emoto's work is popular because of these images, but in essence is providing visual aids of research conducted by several individuals that has been going on for decades, and showing photographic evidence of phenomenon already charted. Visual aids are immeasurably helpful, but do little to answer the how and why, and the answer provided by such photographers to the question "what does this mean" is elementary at best. Proponents and authors such as Emoto seem to primarily focus on the most basic and obvious principle that the photographic phenomenon demonstrates, which is to live one's life with thoughts and intentions of love, thanks, and otherwise positive emotions. This is certainly essential to a positive experience of life and physical, emotional, and spiritual health, but this is by no means a 'new' principle. To live life in love and thanks is as ancient a moral as morals themselves, and one that even Western medicine has subscribed to as being 'good for your health'. It does bring more awareness to the effects negative thoughts or energy frequencies may have on us, and while this is all a great message, it does little to discuss what it *truly means* that water has such amazing structural capacities and that this structure directly relates to our consciousness – a discovery that predates Masaru Emoto's work in the modern era of science and research by more than 20 years.

Today Masaru Emoto might be the most popular name in the public attention surrounding this phenomena, but he is only one among many who have and are researching and demonstrating the properties and effects of consciousness and intention on water, and the effect structured water has on health. Researchers at the HeartMath Research Institute are using spectrophotometers and magnetic resonance imaging (MRI) to examine the effects of healer's hands and magnets, as well as the differences between water from various sacred sites, while other developers are working on structuring and distributing their structured water to individuals on a large scale basis, a challenging task due to water's responsiveness.

Another figure on the forefront of modern structured water science is Dr. Gerald Pollack, a professor of bioengineering from the University of Washington. Dr. Pollack acknowledges that the liquid crystalline phase of Water, i.e. structured water, is much more prevalent than previously thought, and is "intimately connected with the generation and preservation of life."[11] While Marcel Vogel was calling it the "liquid crystal mesophase" in the late 1980's, today Dr. Pollack refers to it as "the fourth phase of water" and is often times inaccurately credited with its discovery (which, like Emoto, also predates Dr. Pollack's work by more than 20 years). To quote Dr. Pollack,

> *The water inside your cells is absolutely critical for your health. If you have a pathology of an organ, it's not only the proteins inside that organ that are not working, but also the water inside that organ. That near-protein water is not ordered in the way in should be. So what you want to do is re-establish a kind of 'ordering'... if you need that entity to function properly – take a muscle for example, if the muscle is not functioning, it's the protein and the water that are not functioning... You need plenty of this ordered/ structured water and proteins in their right form in order to make the muscle function properly. (2011)*

Pollack is absolutely right in that in the instance of pathology, it is not only the proteins that are not functioning, but also the structure of the water. What he does not mention is that the function of the protein

---

11. Pollack, Gerald. *Water, Energy. And Life.* Presented at the 32nd Annual Faculty Lecture, University of Washington, 2009.

is directly dependent upon it being properly structured; that is to say, the protein has to be in the right *shape* in order to work. In the field of intra-cellular biology, it has already been demonstrated that the structure of the *minimum* 10,000 water molecules which surround *every* protein in the body is not just a major factor in determining the shape of that protein, but may even be *directly* responsible for its shape. Since water molecules contain anywhere from 6-300 units of $H_2O$ *per molecule,* we're talking about some 3,000,000 units of $H_2O$ surrounding *every* protein, and sometimes more – water molecules have been observed to surround proteins in even larger numbers than 10,000.

These are the true primary Laws of Physics – the Laws of Structure. These laws are meant not to govern, in the way our traffic laws govern, but rather are meant to merely describe in a logical and coherent form what we consistently observe in nature. The natural order which scientific law seeks to describe does not *cause* anything in nature, the order simply *is,* and everything that naturally occurs is a part of it. The physics and laws demonstrated through structured water science, which involve the laws of patterns and structures, hold vast implications for the potentials of the structure of energy and consciousness. These are the most logical and coherent form of what we consistently observe in nature. Once one understands the true meaning of Water, one realizes there is no greater or more principal Law of Physics than the fundamentals represented in the *structure of energy* and the *structure of water,* particularly the *bio-water,* or the water within our body. It is the fundamental foundation on which all other Laws are based, including both the laws of physics and the laws of meta-physics.

As Western physicists, cellular biologists, and other

scientists slowly come around to acknowledge a fact growing harder to deny with such continuously mounting evidence, researchers in Eastern Europe have taken the study of structured water much farther than most in the United States and Western Europe. Unfortunately, much of it is ignorantly and unjustly criticized and ignored by mainstream science, or is simply unavailable and un-translated. Still, the Russian publications which have been translated (an extremely small percentage of large volumes of work) indicate that their approach to the study of water varies quite differently from published work in the US and Europe, and discusses such aspects of water as its vortexing, superconducting, and energy-generating potentials. As mentioned earlier, Professor Konstantin Korotkov, of the Russian Academy of Natural Sciences (also a Professor of Physics at St. Petersburg, author of over 70 papers in leading journals in physics and biology, and holder of 12 patents in biophysics inventions), has carried out consciousness experiments similar to that of Masaru Emoto. He has also charted other differences in the characteristics of various water samples, i.e. changes in surface tensions, effect on plant growth rates, etc., which exhibit similar differences and results as those charted and observed by *numerous* individuals around the globe. His conclusions, that positive and negative emotions have the largest influence on the structure of water, represents a scientific breakthrough that has until now been largely unrecognized.

*We have carried out many experiments on the effect that quite diverse factors have on samples of water. Magnetic fields, electrical fields, various objects, and also including a human presence, and human emotions. And it became clear that positive and negative human emotions are the strongest element of influence.*

~DR. KONSTANTIN KOROTKOV
DOCTOR OF SCIENCES
PROFESSOR OF PHYSICS
RUSSIAN ACADEMY OF NATURAL SCIENCES

In the Far East, particularly in Japan and Korea, a wide variety of research has also been done on structured and altered water, including water sterilization through exposure to intense magnetic fields, and the biological responses to magnetized water exposed to different frequencies and pulse rates. Dr. Mu Shik Jhon was the President of the Korean Academy of Science and Technology, and the Honorary Chair-Professor of the Korea Advanced Institute of Science and Technology. He was a very prolific scientist with over 250 publications, most of which were published in American scientific journals. Dr. Jhon's research in the realm of structured water, as well as the work of Dr. Yang Oh and Gil-Ho Kim, points to evidence that abnormal water structure in the cellular fluids is directly related to the abnormal cellular activity that results in cancer, diabetes, and AIDS. This water is lacking the geometric complexity and the structural integrity exhibited in the bio-waters of healthy cells, comparable through NMR technology. Nuclear Magnetic Resonance technology is similar to the MRI technologies used in most hospitals, and allows researchers to view the shape, motion, and composition of molecules. NMR examination of cells infected with HIV reveals the same water environment as those with cancer and diabetes – a lack of organized structure at the cellular level.[12]

> ...*cell water is generally different from that of bulk water, and...[becomes] more bulk-like in cancer cells.*
>
> ~PHILLIP BALL
>           20        YEAR          EDITOR: PHYSICAL
>           SCIENCES, INCLUDING    BIOCHEMISTRY AND
>           QUANTUM   PHYSICS, SCIENTIFIC  JOURNAL
>           NATURE

> *The hexagonal structure of water is the one that promotes health and increases longevity.*
> ~DR. YANG H. OH
>           HARVARD GRADUATE
>           RETIRED   BAYLOR   MEDICAL   SCHOOL
>           PROFESSOR

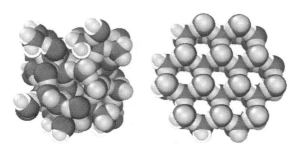

Fig. 3: Left: disorganized molecule arrangement.
Right: organized, or structured, molecule arrangement

12. Dr. Yang Oh and Gil-Ho Kim. *Miracle Molecular Structure of Water.* Pittsburg, PA.: Dorrance Publishing Co., 2002.

42 CARLY NUDAY, PhD

This kind of research is astounding, and proves what Dr. Marcel Vogel knew over 30 years ago and what our ancestors have known throughout antiquity. The implication is clear: the disruption in the cellular activity directly relates to the degradation of the cellular waters – degraded from a highly structured liquid crystalline state to one that is disordered and un-organized, becoming more like bulk water. As this type of research shows, our state of health is dependent upon the structure of our water, and the scientific and medical community will have to contend with this fact eventually. As we will later see when we explore our water system in more depth, the structure of our bodily waters, or *bio-waters*, is part of an integral biofeedback system within our body. The function of both our consciousness and our physical system are both reflective of *and* dependent upon the structure of our bio-waters. Thus, affecting the structure of the water in our body has a direct effect on the function of the physical system, as well as our mental and emotional states. Mainstream science and even "authorities" on water have scoffed at these notions regarding the importance of water's molecular organization and the effect of the dynamic and responsive structural changes it undergoes in response to different stimuli – structural changes that reflect the 'energy' of the stimuli, whether it is an energy that is supportive for life, i.e. 'healthy' or 'positive' energy, or energy that does *not* support life and expresses decay, i.e. 'unhealthy' or 'negative' energy. This phenomenon, while apparently new, actually has a well-documented history within the realm of both modern and ancient discovery, and the evidence that critics are required to ignore in order to avoid the obvious and paramount truth about structured water grows more insurmountable with each passing day.

*Thoughts can change the viscosity of water, it's properties...and changes the effect the water has on a living organism.*
~DR. MARCEL VOGEL

CHAPTER 4

# WATER IS A LIQUID CRYSTAL

---

*What we have found in our laboratory is that the energy of mind projected through a crystal will structure water just like it was frozen into ice. The remarkable and unique differentiation is that, that water, when it is structured with mind and with thought, remains fluid but structured, that type of category is called a liquid crystal, a mesophase, a mesomorphic transition.*
~DR. MARCEL VOGEL

**Definition**: *Liquid Crystal, noun. Main entry date: 1891.* "An organic liquid whose physical properties resemble those of a crystal in the formation of loosely <u>ordered molecular arrays similar to regular crystalline lattice</u> and the anisotropic refraction of light." *Merriam-Webster Dictionary (emphasis added)*

Water is a *Liquid Crystal*. A crystal has atoms and molecules arranged in repeating geometric patterns. Since water is a liquid crystal, rather than a solid-state crystal such as quartz or ruby, it has the ability to change and alter its geometric pattern formation. This means that certain circumstances – namely environment, consciousness, and different energy frequency stimuli (for example, light, sound, and the Schumann Resonance frequency), encourage water to form or change a repeating and geometric pattern of organization and arrangement of its molecules. This is called its *structure*, the way the water molecules pattern and arrange themselves. As a liquid crystal, water uses its various bonding mechanisms to change its order of arrangement, or *lattice structure* (the symmetrical three-dimensional arrangement of atoms inside a crystal), in its flexible response to stimuli and energy of all kinds. These types of bonds include covalent bonds (where atoms share an electron), van der Waals bonds (bonds caused by forces other than covalent bonds, namely electrostatic interactions), and the other apparently unnamed hypothetical bonds that are theorized to account for several of Water's anomalous properties.

Water as a liquid crystal is easily influenced by, or responsive to, stimuli and energy. It changes its pattern to incorporate this new information, that to which it is exposed, and uses these various bonding mechanisms to effectively change its inherent energetic and information content, storage, or 'memory', essentially changing its inherent energetic and information content. Depending on the stimuli or energy to which it was exposed, the structural patterns in the water will change into either higher crystallographic form with greater symmetry and

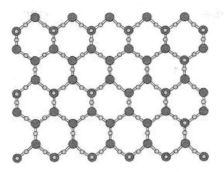

Fig. 4: Example of crystalline
lattice, note repeating geometric
arrangement.

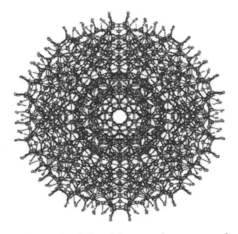

Fig. 5: Organized liquid crystal water molecule
arrangement,
displaying complex geometries.
*Image: Martin Chaplin*
*London South Bank University*

geometric complexity, or it will degrade its structure into
more disorder and display a loss of geometric complexity
and symmetry. Generally speaking, those energies

typically regarded as 'healthy' or 'positive' will improve the water's structure, while those typically regarded as 'unhealthy' or 'negative' will degrade the water's structure. This phenomenon is viewable through the photographic work of Emoto and others, which was previously described, and displays beautiful, complex snowflakes of greater symmetry and organized structure in response to positive intentions and words such as "Love" and "Thank You", but displays misshapen blobs lacking in symmetry, form, and organization when exposed to negative thoughts and words such as "Hate", and harmful artificial electromagnetic frequencies (EMF's) or artificial electromagnetic radiation (EMR), such as those from computers, cell phones, Wi-Fi, and TV's. Misshapen and scattered molecules lacking form are considered de-structured water, while structured water refers to water that exists in its liquid crystalline state, and displays organized and repeating geometric structures, to varying degrees of complexity, in its atomic and molecular formations.

Why does this matter? Because this molecular organization changes the water's properties – making it a vastly different substance than 'bulk' water, the random arrangements of molecules we are taught exist in every glass and every cell. It matters because the specific organization of the water's structure directly relates to the storage and conduction of energy and information within our bodies – because our bodies are made mostly of Structured Water. By molecular content, (rather than mass weight), we are over 99% structured water. This means when we count the number of molecules in our body, we find that over **99% of our molecules are highly structured and crystallographic water.**

This fact is remarkable, and completely changes the

way we view our bodies and our health. Our current paradigm of physiology and biology, of electro-chemical processes, and of aging and disease, has to be completely reworked from this point of view. Water molecules are so small and weigh so little, that while they only comprise 75-80% of our mass weight, they account for over 99% of our molecules. *We are made of over 99% structured water – literally, truly, and scientifically water beings as much as human beings.* If we are to understand how our bodies work, and thus understand our health and wellness, we *must* begin to understand our true water system. Our water system is composed of structured water rather than bulk water, which are nearly two completely different substances. Thus, our knowledge of what structured water really is suddenly becomes critically important if we are to truly understand the actions and implications of 99% of our molecules. And with 99% of our body being structured water, it suddenly becomes critically important if we are to understand ourselves at all.

CHAPTER 5

# THE IMPORTANCE OF
# STRUCTURE

---

*Since the molecular structure of water is the essence of all Life, the
man who can control that structure in cellular systems will change the
world.*
~DR. ALBERT SZENT-GYORGYI
NOBEL PRIZE PHYSIOLOGY OR MEDICINE

*The beauty of a living thing is not the atoms that go into it, it's the
way those atoms are put together.*
~CARL SAGAN
ASTROPHYSICIST

Throughout fields of science everywhere, it is
becoming much more widely understood that what is
critical about *any* substance, and what makes it 'do what
it does', whether it be water, proteins, gold, or even DNA,
has much *less* to do with what elements or compounds it
is actually composed of, and much *more* to do with the
importance of its *structural formation*. This means that it is

CARLY NUDAY, PhD

*not* the chemical ingredients that are important; it is the *shape* and *structure* of the entire unit.

For example, you can replace all of the amino-acids comprising a protein while retaining its molecular formation, essentially making it the *same shape,* like a piece of jigsaw puzzle cut the right way but with the wrong color paint on it, now essentially a 'non-sensical' protein. Theoretically, the body would not know what to do with such a random arrangement of ingredients. If our bodies worked like our eyes do with jigsaw puzzles, the piece wouldn't make any sense no matter how perfectly it fit. But because *everything* is truly structurally based, the body *does* know what to do with it, and the protein will continue to function as if it had the previously arranged information, i.e. the right colored paint on the jigsaw puzzle. It turns out that the information is *not* stored in the protein's actual *ingredients* or its chemical composition. In the jigsaw puzzle of life, the color paint or the picture it creates means *nothing* – as long as the pieces fit perfectly together. With the protein experiment, we see that it had nothing to do with which amino acids the protein contained – *all* of the protein's information was stored in its *structure.* It did not matter what it was made out of, as long as its key fit the lock. What is important are the pattern, shape, and structure. **This rule seems to apply *everywhere.***

*Their theory was that the chemical composition is important. Now the sensational news is that that is nonsense. The structure of the water is much more important than the chemical composition.*
~RUSTUM ROY
PROFESSOR, UNIVERSITY OF
PENNSYLVANIA

MEMBER: INTERNATIONAL ACADEMY
OF SCIENCE

Crystals have unique ways they arrange their atoms and molecules, called the molecular and atomic structures of *crystallographic patterns*. It is these various crystallographic patterns that give rise to their remarkable properties, and it is these symmetrical crystallographic patterns that structured water also expresses. While many are perhaps unfamiliar with the term *liquid crystal*, and discussions of 'atomic and molecular structural formation,' viewing their expression in solid-state crystals can help one to easily grasp the importance of this concept. In the world of crystals, it is easy to see why structure is important.

Each type of crystal – be it diamond, emerald, ruby, quartz, etc. – has a specific structural pattern of molecular arrangement. In fact, it is this arrangement that determines whether a substance is a crystal at all, and it is the number one pre-requisite for placement in this category. If a substance has a repeating geometric pattern of molecular arrangement – a 3 dimensional grid of symmetrically arranged molecules, called a *lattice formation* – then it is called a *crystal*. As a crystal grows, or becomes changed or crystallized due to different forces (pressure, heat, etc.), the atoms become arranged in a specific pattern and display a geometric form of structural organization. This specific pattern arrangement also determines the characteristics and properties of the said crystal: how it will react to light, heat, pressure, UV rays, and other sources of energy and stimuli. The way light or energy, for example, will be conducted or moved through a crystal, depends on how the molecules are arranged. The *structure* determines the *properties.*

Take Carbon, for example. There's Carbon in the form of Graphite, and then there is *Crystalline Carbon,* known as *Diamonds.* Graphite and Diamond might share the same chemical composition – Carbon – but they are drastically different substances, ask any woman. In graphite, the carbon arranges itself in flat sheets stacked on top of each other, and thus is brittle and breaks easily as in pencil lead. The carbon in diamonds knits itself together so perfectly, a 3 dimensional interlocking grid of perfect symmetry and form, that it becomes the hardest substance on Earth. The same follows for the Silicon Dioxide ($SiO_2$) family, which exists as Flint, Glass ('amorphous', or 'unstructured'), and Quartz (*Crystalline SiO_2)* – and while you cannot make a watch, radio, or hard drive out of flint or glass, quartz is largely responsible for our entire technological era. These are just a few examples of the importance of *crystalline structures.* It is the Laws of Structure that allows for substances to be comprised of the same elemental ingredients, varying only in their *patterns of structure,* to create very different substances with very different properties. It is these properties that have allowed both Earth and mankind to evolve, and on which our societies and lives depend. Through these examples we see quite clearly that comparing bulk, unorganized water to structured water is like comparing graphite, or even coal, which is carbon even less organized than graphite, to diamonds. If we are made of diamonds – or at least the $H_2O$ equivalent – it becomes quite ludicrous to approach the body and our health as if it is a system made of graphite or coal.

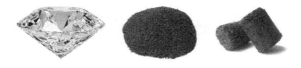

Fig. 6: Diamond, graphite, and coal, all made of
carbon.
The difference is in the structure.

While water exists as solid-state crystal (ice), its responsiveness to certain stimuli – *which causes it to rearrange its structural pattern and thus change its properties*, is because of its amazing ability as a **liquid crystal**. Water with its molecular formations arranged in crystalline lattice formations, i.e. geometric arrangements, goes by many names and is being marketed all over the world. This Water is often called structured, hexagonal, organized, sacred, holy, hydrogenated, oxygenated, magnetized, alkaline, enhanced, clustered, living water, etc.

*Liquid Crystals* are flexible, and can re-pattern their arrangement nearly instantly with new information from stimuli, the characteristic responsible for the phenomenon witnessed in the Emoto and Korotkov photographic experiments. The molecules of liquid crystalline water remain mobile while moving together in their pattern of organization, much like a perfectly orchestrated school of fish. They can, and in the case of water often do, rearrange themselves in *femtoseconds* (one-quadrillionth of a second) and *picoseconds* (one-trillionth of a second) to form a new pattern of structural organization. Every time water rearranges itself, it is encoding new information in the structure while still remaining a highly intelligently organized and mobile 'school of molecular fish'. This flexibility and mobility makes liquid crystals many more times responsive than solid-state crystals. *This responsiveness is one of the most important attributes of water, and is what allows it to have 'memory', able to store energy and charge of specific natures, while also allowing it to update its pattern with the new information to which it is exposed – expressing an intelligence and learning ability.* Rearranging its structure every femtosecond or picosecond does not imply an entirely *new* pattern or base form of organization, but rather an *updating* of its current structural energy.

> *[Structured Water] may be the single most malleable computer.*
> ~ RUSTUM ROY

Rustum Roy called it a "malleable computer" because Water can function as an operating system, has a storage capacity, and it is constantly updating its system. These facts become very important when discussing our real water system in our body, how it operates, and what information it is storing.

The molecular arrangements in structured water display crystallographic, geometric complexity to varying degrees, from extremely dense and complex arrangements to simple and basic geometric patterns. These changes in structure cause dramatic changes in water's property, and are responsible for its anomalous behavior. These changes of the scientifically observed "anomalous" properties for structured water include higher surface tension, changes in freezing temperature and pH, increases in its ORP (Oxidizing Reduction

Potential), geometric organization causing changes in ice crystal formation, greater molecular stability and molecular alignment, an enhanced ability to absorb certain spectra of light, negative electrical charge, greater mineral solubility, greater oil solubility, and micro-clustering (wherein molecules are arranged in smaller groups, allowing for better cellular penetration and thus hydration).

The above examples are just a few of the measured physical changes of properties that have been observed, and such changes in properties are extremely important for all of Life's processes – which depend not just on water, but on *structured water* to support all of its great diversity of forms and flora. Changes in pH, which indicates the amount of hydrogen in a liquid, means it is better for life-supporting systems, which require a slightly alkaline (rather than acidic) environment for health. A greater oxidizing reduction potential (O.R.P.) simply means its ability to donate energy to the body through its hydrogen atoms, which donates electrical charge (as in "anti-oxidant") in the form of electrons to free radical oxygen. Larger absorption of certain spectra of light, as well as greater negative electrical charge (i.e. ionization) means the water holds greater energy potential and is more conductive than un-organized, or bulk water, its conductive nature being critical to Life's every process. Greater mineral and oil solubility means better delivery of necessary nutrients to cells. Micro-clustering causes better penetration through the aquaporin channels in the body through smaller molecules, making it easier to bring nutrients to the cell, toxins out of the cell, and is said to be three times more hydrating than larger clusters of water molecules.

The structure of the water in our body (our bio-water)

and its properties are vital to the existence, function, and maintenance of our body, brain, and bio-energetic systems. The level of structure, or the degree of how geometrically precise and complex the arrangement of molecules, has a direct effect on the level of function and energetic capacities of both the bio-water and our physical and energetic systems.

*I have put now almost 27 years of study into this type of structure. It is organized, it is holding information and it takes the minutest charge to release it and make it to come back to its normal water bulk characteristic. We speak of vital water, we speak of holy water, we speak of Lourdes water, we speak of the sacred springs, and each one of these statements I find to be true. When I have studied waters from various sacred locales, I find a structure in that water which is unique from the bulk water... I have found waters that test 40,000 times more energetic than bulk water... These should not even be considered the same substance.*

~DR. MARCEL VOGEL
IBM SCIENTIST, CRYSTALLOGRAPHER

# PART II

# WATER MECHANICS: THE TRUE LAWS OF NATURE

*The greatest impediment to scientific innovation is usually a conceptual lock, not a factual lack.*
~STEPHEN JAY GOULD
HARVARD PALEONTOLOGIST

Exactly *how* Water is able to exhibit such phenomena and remarkable changes in properties and structure has until now largely remained a mystery. To understand how water achieves such incredible phenomena, we must have a basic understanding of the principles on which it operates, which include specific geometric patterns of information, energy, and fractality (the concept of shapes which can be split apart into parts, each of which is an approximate reduced-sized copy of the whole, where the parts express self-similar patterns viewable at greater and greater magnifications, i.e. the branching ends of snowflakes, or the intricate nesting of rose petals), as well as the ability to translate entropic and non-entropic energetic information into physical expression. If these words are completely new to you, don't worry – they will be defined in the following sections. These statements, when read with an understanding for the definition of their terms, will reveal large implications about the abilities and mechanics of water as we explore them. Water, so critical to Universal Life, reveals incredible magic about the way energy and consciousness operate in our reality, magic that remains hidden until we understand the way Water itself operates, reflecting as the original mirror the marvelous dynamics of our existence.

CHAPTER 6

# THE STRUCTURES IN CRYSTALS
# AND WATER

---

## DEFINING FREQUENCIES, COHERENCE, AND RESONANCE

Water, as a liquid crystal, orders its molecular arrangement into crystalline lattice formations. These are, essentially, repeated angles, vectors (specific mathematical structures and lines), vertices (points of angles, where lines intersect), and geometries, or mathematical shapes. By examining the study of crystallography, through which a great deal about geometric patterns is known, we can understand much about the importance of the structure of water. Both liquid and solid crystal patterns vary in their mathematical geometries and symmetries, and *these geometric patterns are expressions of the energetic information they contain.* Thus, their specific crystal structures determine their properties, or characteristics and abilities, their "memory" and responsive information storage, and their ability to transmit signals, as organized patterns provide efficient pathways for the flow of energetic information. This applies to both liquid and solid-state crystals.

The fact that solid-state crystalline structures are able to both store and transmit information is a property, or ability, used by modern society since before the original crystal radios. Remember when computers were the size of a large room or a small house? It was the development of the quartz crystal based computer chips and microprocessors that have made computers what they are today, thanks to their ability to transfer and process information. Today we know that crystals also have *enormous* potential for storage and archival information, and we have just begun to scratch the surface of their abilities to hold immense amounts of data. For example, in Hamburg, Tennessee, scientists have already successfully stored and retrieved thousands of 3D holographic images *from a single niobate crystal,* which are typically only inches in diameter.[1] In Japan, the electronics giant Hitachi and Kyoto University are laser-etching information into slivers of quartz that can preserve information for hundreds of millions of years without degrading, or breaking down. These quartz chips are also waterproof and resistant to chemicals and weathering, including temperatures exceeding 1,000°C in testing, and have thus been dubbed "Superman crystals". We know that entire library databases, including the entire Library of Congress, can be stored onto a single crystal. And in today's technology world, if not for cloud-based storage systems, we would almost certainly be using quartz storage systems in our everyday computers. Crystals can potentially last nearly forever, as their molecules are so symmetrically arranged that they don't 'break down' like normal materials, a process sometimes referred to as *entropy.* With this type of nearly permanent lifespan and their capacity and efficiency for information storage and retrieval, quartz hard drives would have been developed to replace the current crystalline iron

1. Gerber, Richard, M.D. 2001.

'magnetite' based hard drive systems of today (originally developed by Dr. Marcel Vogel), if not for our recent increase in use and development of storing information in "the cloud", i.e. storing it online. These capabilities, from watches and radios, to computer chips, computer screens, and database storage, are only made possible by the patterns, and thus the properties, of crystalline structures.

The geometric structures of the molecular arrangement in crystals that allow them to record so much information are the same geometric structures that are responsible for water's phenomenal memory recording. It has been recorded, for example, that each group of water molecules, called a *cluster*, works as a type of "memory cell". These clusters vary in size and complexity, containing up to hundreds and even a thousand molecules, but most commonly observed in groups of 3-60 molecules and expressing various types and degrees of geometric patterns. Some have recorded there to be at least 440,000 different 'panels' of information storage within *each* cluster, or memory cell.[2] Having acknowledged that solid-state crystals have vast potentials for information storage, from the 3-D images in Hamburg to the potentials of entire library databases, it is not difficult to grasp that the same geometric structures present in water as a liquid crystal allow it the same property of information storage.

Crystalline structures can also cause the *coherence of*

2. *Water, the Great Mystery.* Dir. Anastasiya Popova. Intention Media Inc., 2008. Documentary Film.

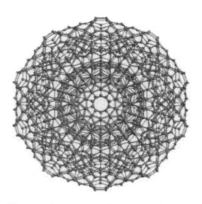

Fig. 7: Structured water cluster
model.
*Image: Martin Chaplin*
*London South Bank University*

*energy transmission*, wherein the energy projected through
its structure becomes correlated, synchronized, or in
phase with one another. *Coherence* is a property that is
most easily seen in observing the action of light in ruby
crystals, and can be understood by comparing
incandescent bulbs to lasers. With incandescent bulbs, the
light emitted is scattered randomly in all directions, and
is thus *incoherent* light. Light projected through a properly
cut ruby, however, will cohere the light – focusing the
light waves in one direction and projecting them as
synchronized, *cohered* waves, all moving together, thus
creating the original laser. The electromagnetic energy
waves need not be of the same *frequency* in order to be
coherent. Frequencies that are *harmonic*, meaning they
have a complimentary mathematical relationship – like
harmonic musical notes in a chord – may still operate
or vibrate in coherence with one another, having found
synchronization in a harmonic scale. A laser exhibits this

synchronized wave emission – also called coherence.

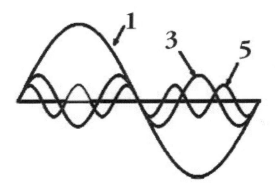

Fig. 8: Energy Coherence and Harmonics.
These waves are in perfect mathematical ratios,
repeating exactly 3 and 5 times within the
sequence of the larger primary wave. These waves
are coherent: in phase, harmony, and
synchronization with each other.

Let us further define and demonstrate these concepts, for they are fundamental principles. As previously discussed, a *frequency* is a specific electromagnetic or energy wave pattern. In mainstream science, it applies only to electromagnetic activity, since there is not yet an appropriate understanding of the mechanics of subtle energy (also called 'magneto-electric' energy), a topic we will explore later. Yet science has long recognized that all electrical activity has a corresponding magnetic field, and all magnetic fields have a corresponding electrical value, thus energy is at once both *electric* and *magnetic* in nature and is hence termed *electromagnetic*. The electromagnetic energy waves have specific patterns, which are measured as its frequency. Frequencies are incredibly important, and a primary mechanism our Universe uses in its expression. Everything – from cells, tissue groups, organs, systems, and individuals, to different atomic elements and compounds of matter, are all emitting electromagnetic frequencies, different patterns of energy that are unique to its source – i.e. its vibrational signature. Every element on the periodic table emits its own specific electromagnetic frequency signature, as does the Earth, which emits a harmonic chord of fluctuating frequencies most often resonating at 7-8 Hertz, or Hz, the term used for measuring electromagnetic waves. Electromagnetic waves are emitting from every organism and object, every atom and molecule, every star, and every planet. They are all sound and light waves, radio waves, microwaves, and x-rays. These waves of electromagnetic energy are assigned a value of frequency based on the speed at which the wave travels, and how many times the peak of the oscillation, or vibrating wave, moves past a point each second. Thus, a certain note or sound has a frequency (measured in Hertz, or Hz, which can be taken literally to mean "cycles per second", as in how many times the wave repeats its pattern in a single second), as does a certain color of light (typically measured in *wavelengths*, as opposed to the Hz system of cycles per second, as light travels much faster than sound and has a much higher Hz value), or the certain frequency of a radio station or cell phone (often referred to as harmful artificial electromagnetic radiation and frequencies, or EMR and EMF, respectively, which are often vibrating in the 'microwave' range of the electromagnetic spectrum). The 7 Hz frequency used in the Montagnier experiment discussed earlier, then, is an electromagnetic wave that repeats its pattern 7 times in one second. On the electromagnetic scale, audible sound and voice frequencies are between 20 and 20,000 Hz for the average human, while for dogs it ranges between 40 and 60,000 Hz. Visible light waves are much faster than audible sound, and range between 430 and 790 Tera-hertz, or trillions of cycles per second for humans. Because they are in the trillions of hertz, light waves are usually measured in terms of *nanometers*. Several species of birds, insects, and reptiles perceive visible light waves in the ultra-violet (UV-light) side of the scale, outside human visual perception. Power lines are operating at a certain frequency, as are radio waves, cell-phones, and Wi-Fi signals – all emitting a specific band, or range, of frequencies. We are constantly receiving incoming energy in the form of electromagnetic frequencies, information both perceivable to our senses (i.e. visual light, sound), and not perceivable to our senses (i.e. the electromagnetic frequency waves emitted by cell phones, radio signals, power lines, etc.). The specific electromagnetic frequency will carry certain information in its wave and frequency pattern – whether that information is perceivable by our senses, i.e. light waves in the color 'red', or is not perceivable, i.e. the electromagnetic frequency waves emitted by a cell phone. Consciously perceived or not, our cells, tissue groups, organs, water, and system as a whole receives and reacts to incoming electromagnetic frequencies. All forms of modern science and biology acknowledge this fact, while the subject of *how* the body is influenced, either positively or negatively by such various electromagnetic frequencies, is much less well understood.

The human body has a complex electromagnetic system, as information is transferred among systems via electromagnetic frequencies, and electromagnetic frequencies play a large part in cellular communication and processes. In the cellular world, much activity happens by way of electromagnetic frequencies, and in fact not a single reaction happens in the body that is not *electro-magnetic* in nature, meaning that every reaction in the body uses electromagnetic energy in order to work. In the body, there is no such thing as a 'bio-chemical reaction', there are only 'electro-bio-chemical reactions'. Cells use electromagnetic energy to send signals, to open and close cellular ports, and in fact to successfully create *every* cellular process. Electromagnetic signals are used to induce cascades of physical reactions in the body, and even for the body to communicate with its environment. The electromagnetic field of the heart, for example, is incredibly strong and is detectable even 60 feet away from the human body with rather simple equipment. Every cell in the body is actively registering and transferring all energy within its environment, and is constantly initiating an appropriate response based on how it translates the incoming frequency information.

> *Cells can recognize extremely subtle differences in electric fields, noting their waveforms, amplitudes, and frequencies. They then decode them, decide how to respond, and initiate a response... Cells also recognize other communications, other languages from the environment... this sensitivity to subtle communications in the electromagnetic spectrum is not limited to cells. Even enzymes and molecules recognize and process different electromagnetic frequencies... These kinds of oscillations, or wave signals, make up one of the primary languages used by all self-organized systems.*
> ~STEPHEN HARROD BUHNER

The electromagnetic energy field of an individual is a *complex harmonic of nested frequencies*, wherein every cell emits a frequency, and groups of cells synchronize their vibrations to either match frequencies or vibrate in tune, or resonance – that is, in phase, in sync, or in harmony together. Viewed from the mathematical perspective, these waves will be in a balanced relationship, and the level of balance may even indicate the level of the body's health. Wave harmonics can be easily viewed through music, where octaves of the same note represent an equal relationship in the ratio of their frequencies. For example, the low 'C' note on the piano has a frequency of 16.35 Hz – repeating its wave pattern cycle 16.35 times in one second. Eight notes, or one octave higher, we find again the 'C' note, only of a higher pitch – this one vibrating at 32.7 Hz, or twice as fast as the lower octave C. The next 'C' on the piano has a frequency of 65.41 Hz, vibrating four times as fast as the lower C and twice as fast as the octave before it. When the relationship of the frequency is a precise ratio, as with octaves, it is what we call a 'harmonic vibration'. The average ear can easily recognize the difference between harmonic chords of music and dissonant or 'out of tune' chords – out of tune because they do not resonate, or vibrate, at harmonious frequencies of complimenting wave patterns.

The human body operates on incredibly complex harmonies of nested electromagnetic information, frequencies emitted from individual cells, groups of cells, enzymes, bacteria, organs, the brain, the frequencies generated by the movement of blood and fluids, bone, etc. What this means is that all of these different frequencies are woven together, much like musical notes in a chord. Thus we cannot assign one particular frequency to an individual, as various parts of the body resonate with different frequencies, all projecting energy which when combined becomes the electromagnetic field of the person, a dynamic and constantly adjusting energetic field. The heart alone is a strong and complex electromagnetic generator. It is not a singular frequency but a group of frequencies, created by each cell and cell group, as well as the movement of action and pulsing, and the electrical and magnetic activity of the organ, and the electromagnetic energy generated by the blood moving inside of it. These numerous different frequencies and energy waves are woven together like a nest, or fitted together like a nesting doll, stacked inside of or on top of each other in perfectly fitting ratios. The body, in ideal health, is resonating frequencies of cells, tissue groups, and organs that are all synchronized in harmonic mathematical ratios.

This harmonic vibration allows for *coherency within the system* – where information can be gathered, translated, relayed, and received in the most productive and efficient manner possible. We engage in electromagnetic communication and information transfer every day as we emit electromagnetic frequencies from our heart, brain, and body *into* our environment, and receive electromagnetic frequencies through our heart, brain, and body *from* our environment. Frequencies are used in the body to react to changes in the internal or external environment, such as temperature, weather, and time of day, and for translating electromagnetic information into various forms, such as the photoreceptors and audio receptors which translate certain frequencies into their respective perceived sound or light. We are impacted by frequencies of electromagnetic energy that are not even perceivable to us – already we described the Schumann Resonance of the Earth's natural electromagnetic frequency and the way an individual's health rapidly deteriorates when denied exposure to this field.

Frequency then, can be understood as a *specific pattern of radiating energy*, descriptive of its speed, type, or intensity of energy, perceivable or not perceivable. We mentioned previously that the body, in ideal health, is resonating the combined frequencies of all of its cells, tissue groups, and organs in synchronized and harmonic mathematical ratios, as this harmonic vibration allows for *coherency within the system* – where information can be gathered, translated, relayed, and received in the most productive and efficient manner possible. From this perspective, disease could really be considered *dissonance*, where some pathology of a system or symptom of disorder would be reflective in its vibrations, oscillations, or frequencies being out of phase or out of tune, deviating from its normal, healthy pattern and causing *incoherence* within the system.

Coherence, when used this way in physics, is defined as: "pertaining to waves that maintain a fixed phase relationship" or relating to "two or more waves having the same phase or a fixed phase difference." A fixed phase difference or relationship refers to the harmonic ratios described earlier, using the example of multiple musical notes of a chord – a harmonic chord of music vibrates multiple sounds into one resonant group of vibrations, rather than a dissonant cord where the multiple sounds do not blend in a coherent nested manner but rather produce a jarring sound readily recognized by the ears and body. Thus, another definition for *coherent* is "having a natural agreement of parts; harmonious."

When discussing *coherence* among multiple frequencies, we are also talking about the *organization and synchronization of information and energy* – the more coherence in a system, the more organization there is, which means more information and more energy can be contained and transferred. This property of coherence is easily viewed through the *coherence of brainwave patterns.* Here, measurements taken using EEG devices can measure electrical impulses emitted by different regions of the brain, and determine their level of synchronization and rhythm. States of meditation are associated with an increase in brainwave coherence. Higher rates and patterns of coherence are also associated with more integrated and effective thinking and behavior, which often express as greater intelligence, creativity, learning abilities, emotional stability, self-confidence, and reduced anxiety, as well as other traits and expressions we would normally regard as 'healthy' or 'positive'. This is also viewed in the measurable coherence of the heart rate and its emissions, wherein greater coherence has been associated with a longer life span, a healthier and higher functioning physiology, greater emotional wellness, a stronger immune system, higher quality of life, and an increase in the effectiveness of communication between cells and systems.

In terms of electromagnetic energy, particularly when discussing the frequencies of an individual or their brainwave patterns, *coherence* is as important as *frequency.* The different frequency bandwidths exhibited by the brain relate to its electrical energy and are associated with brain activity, but the level of *coherence* reflects the amount of information in the system. For example, Mozart was operating at the same bandwidths of brainwave frequencies as everyone else, but likely had a much higher level of *coherence* within his frequencies, with certain regions of his brain oscillating or vibrating at specific rates and emitting electromagnetic waves that had a specific harmonious relationship to each other. These frequency emissions, based on the individual's brain activity, in a coherent system, are woven together in a synchronized pattern, creating smaller and more complex unique patterns within the larger context of its measured brain wave frequency pattern – patterns called *fractals,* which transfer and store *massive* amounts of information.

Let us consider this further, to build our understanding and really grasp this fundamental reality and principle of energetic physics. As we have already discussed, every cell emits a wave pattern, or frequency. In a state of health, groups of cells, each emitting an individual pattern of energy waves, synchronize their wave emissions, or vibrations, to vibrate in harmony, in synchronization, in rhythm, and in *coherence.* Each wave pattern, when magnified, reveals smaller patterns within its larger structure, patterns that are self-similar, i.e. similar to its larger 'parent' pattern. Each time the magnification is increased, it reveals smaller and smaller patterns that are yet still similar to its larger structure. These are called *fractals,* and are easy to see in the branching ends of snowflakes, which become smaller and smaller versions of an overall larger pattern. In a *coherent* system, where the wave patterns are vibrating in harmony with one another, these different patterns combine to make intricate, complex, and unique geometries. In a coherent system, the geometries that are created from the weaving and combining of different frequency patterns of energy are *precise* in their shape and angles. The intersecting lines and structure, or *vectors,* of the geometric patterns that are created have specific angles – where points and lines intersect and cross, creating edges, definitive points in the patterns, and exacting angles – also called *vertices* and *vertexes.* From a physics perspective, the *vertices,* or angles, are where information is actually present and stored, and the lines between the angles, or *vectors,* are typically viewed as the directional paths on which information travels throughout the network. The *vertices,* or angles, which store information are also sometimes called *nodal points,* as they are essentially points at which lines or pathways intersect at a connecting point in the network.

In a *coherent system,* such as that displayed by Mozart's musical brain, each of the different groups of cells, or different areas of the brain, emit different energy wave patterns in synchronized harmony, which intersect with each other and form geometric shapes within their vibrating energy wave patterns. These geometric patterns are complex, unique, and store and transfer large amounts of information in the energetic dialogue that occurs between all interacting waveforms of energy.

This is essentially the magic and power behind a coherent energy system. *Coherence* – synchronized wave patterns – brings *geometric nested fractality,* i.e. complex patterns of nested and woven geometric patterns which, when magnified, reveal even smaller and smaller similar patterns within their structures. This in turn translates into exponential increases in the information transfer and capabilities of the system. These unique frequency patterns, with their complex and intricate weaving or nesting of the many frequencies emitted by the brain (and body) are creating fractal geometries, these self-similar sub-units, or smaller and smaller 'patterns within the pattern', and within its coherent expression of all of these synchronized waves. This allows for a great amount of information transfer and processing within the system, thus Mozart, with a high level of specific frequency coherence, had the ability to recognize frequencies, waves, and their relationships, and applied this to music, integrating patterns and harmonies in ways most people could never dream of. Using EEG monitors, which register the different electromagnetic signals from various areas of the brain, we can now measure brainwave coherence, and see in a visual representation the synchronized or non-synchronized wave patterns. The image on the following page displays the effect that Transcendental Meditation®, a specific type of meditation practice, has on brainwave coherence. The first image displays EEG readings from a non-meditating subject, while the second displays a subject during Transcendental Meditation®. Not only is there more brain *activity* during Transcendental Meditation®, there is also greater *coherence* and synchronization throughout the system. Meditation practices of all kinds are known to improve brainwave coherence, and the EEG scans of the meditating subject, who is experiencing a high state of brainwave coherence at the time of the scan, give us a graphic representation of the increase in the *complex geometric nesting of patterns of energy* (Fig. 9).

When one considers the actual physical reality of what is occurring in the brain at any given time, we see that there are streams of different types of electromagnetic energy, different frequencies and patterns of energy emitting from all areas of the brain simultaneously. Simultaneously does not necessarily mean synchronized, nor does it mean complexly organized. However, we see the synchronization and complexity of activity in *all* areas of the brain increases *dramatically* when a person is meditating. These energy patterns, their level of complexity and organization, determine the capabilities of the system. How much information can a person's brain retrieve, process, store, and transfer, and how complex can the information be? These questions are answered by the level of coherence within the system.

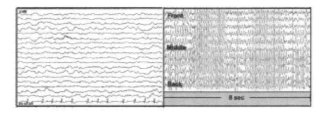

Fig. 9: Brain Coherence.
Left: Typical EEG tracings from non-meditating subject.
Right: EEG tracings recorded from subject while practicing Transcendental Meditation® techniques.
Image: Travis, Fred. "A Self-Referential Default Brain State."
Cognitive Processing 11.1(2010):21-30.

Electromagnetic energy waves are dynamic, and as we further explore the importance of patterns, geometry, and fractality, we will see even more clearly what is happening behind the veil of coherent energies. The level of coherence within the system allows for complex information retrieval, processing, storage, and transfer because the different electromagnetic frequencies express complex geometries within their own pattern, and interact with each other's various complex geometries to nest and combine, in a matching and synchronized rhythm, creating even *more* intricate geometric patterns in their energetic dialogue and exchange of information.

One of the reasons incredible things happen when coherence occurs is the *resonance wave.* We discussed resonance earlier by describing one of the ways the word is used – to indicate a resonating wave, as in its reverberations, or emitted vibrations. Another way it is often used is actually similar to coherence; when two or more frequencies are vibrating in phase, coherence, nested or in harmonious mathematical ratios with each other, they are referred to as having *resonance,* which is really an expression of coherence. Then there is the principle of Resonance, which encompasses also the phenomena of the *resonance wave.* This principle refers to the way in which the vibrations of one thing affect the vibrations of another – causing it to change its vibrations of electromagnetic energy in order to oscillate at a frequency that will be in phase, or resonance, with the original dominating vibration. This principle can be easily seen in the action of tuning forks, which are designed to vibrate at a specific frequency. If one has two tuning forks tuned to the same pitch, or frequency, in the same room, they need only to strike one of the tuning forks to get them both to vibrate. Here the Principle of Resonance is readily apparent – the vibrating waves of one thing are used to affect the vibrations of another. Because of the *resonance* between the two tuning forks, the vibrating wave emissions of the first tuning fork, upon reaching the second tuning fork, causes it to also vibrate. Another example happens between strings of musical instruments, even those of different notes, as long as they share a harmonic octave – for example, a string tuned to the A note of 440 Hz will also cause an E string at 330 Hz to resonate, or vibrate, because they share an overtone, or a harmonic pitch of their octaves at 1320 Hz (the 3rd harmonic, or octave of A and the 4th harmonic, or octave, of E). The Principle of Resonance can also be seen by the actions of the opera singer who, when vocalizing at the right pitch (or specific sound frequency) breaks a glass: the frequency of the pitch causes the vibrations of the glass to speed up, trying to achieve resonance with the vibrations of the sound, eventually the molecules of the glass are no longer able to retain their original structure with the increased energy and change in frequency, thus the glass shatters and the energy is released. This is an example of when resonance is *not* achieved – the molecules of glass cannot vibrate at so high a frequency and still remain 'glass'. When the principle of Resonance *is* achieved between two frequencies, however, and two waves become synchronized, harmonious, in phase, and *coherent*, and here we observe the phenomenon of the appearance of a *new* wave, outside of the original two frequencies, a new wave which can now be detected in the pattern. This new wave is really the magic of the synergy that occurs in achieved resonance, wherein coherent resonance is achieved, energy and information is transferrable, and something new is created. In the realm of the principle of Resonance, coherence, and the resonant wave, one plus one really does equal three. This is the very definition of synergy, where the result is greater than the sum of its parts. This resonance wave also represents the energetic dialogue when resonance is achieved – the information transfer between two systems that creates new information based on their communication. Let us view this through the lens of human nature, where resonance can easily be seen through a successful relationship. Two individuals, coming together and having resonance, establish a third wave of energy, that which comes out of their relationship, the energetic dialogue between them in constant exchange, constantly creating new information, viewed as the growth and fruits of their relationship, the synergy that is created from the coming together of these two separate individuals.

Frequency, Coherence, and Resonance are important principles and terms to understand when discussing electromagnetic energy, particularly as it relates to crystals, water, and physiology. Using principles of resonance, the vibrating frequencies of one thing can be used to affect the vibrating frequencies of another thing and can be used to establish coherence between the two systems, thus increasing the amount, quality, and efficiency of informational processing. This has been viewed using EEG scans and other monitoring devices to observe changes in brainwave patterns during intentional or subtle energy healings, where conscious energy from one individual is used to affect the health and mental state to stimulate healing in another. Changes in the brainwave patterns of the 'healer' have been observed to fluctuate and change until there is a level of resonance established between the brainwave patterns of the 'healer' and the 'healee', at which point the brainwave patterns of the 'healer' begin to fluctuate and raise to a more coherent frequency pattern, and in effect are able to bring the brainwave frequencies of the 'healee' into a more stable frequency pattern and greater coherence at the same time through the established resonance.[3] This is how the actual healing is achieved, as having a more stable frequency pattern and greater coherence greatly affects if not determines our level of health.

As both liquid crystals (i.e. water) and solid-state crystals (i.e. quartz) are both part of the crystalline family, there is an inherent level of *sympathy* between these two systems, which is largely responsible for the effect crystals have been observed to have on the structure of water. The use of solid-state crystals is one of the primary methods used to bring about liquid crystallographic structural changes in water, the details of which will be

3. Gerber, Richard, M.D. 2001.

further explored later on as we discuss different structuring methods.

The effects solid-state crystals have on electromagnetic energy are astounding. It is largely because of this fact that we have been able to advance our technological developments, from the original crystal-based radios and quartz watches to today's microchips and advanced computing crystal based systems. In addition to their incredible memory and storage capabilities, and their ability to cohere frequencies (such as the laser light of a properly cut ruby), they are also able to *amplify, transmute, transform, transfer, transmit, and transduce* electromagnetic energy. They can cause energy to change forms or be conducted, emit energy of high forms and frequency, and release energy through their resonating frequencies. These abilities can be observed through remarkable properties many crystals express, such as *piezoelectricity* (mechanical pressure resulting in electrical energy, i.e. quartz, bone, etc.) *pyroelectricity* (applied heat resulting in electrical energy), *birefringence* (the splitting of a light ray into 2 separate light rays, perpendicular to each other), *semi-conductivity* (the ability to conduct energy and information without resistance or loss of information within the system), *infrared emissions* (crystals which emit frequency waves and vibrations in the infrared portion of the electromagnetic spectrum), *ionizations* (crystals which release negatively charged particles into the atmosphere, donating energy in the form of negative ions), *radiation emissions* (the emission of energy waves which carry electrical charge), *pyroluminosity* (applied heat causing phosphorescence), etc. All of these attributes relate to the ability of crystalline structures to transform and transduce energy. The different properties attributed to different classes or types of crystals relates to their differences in geometric atomic and molecular arrangement and structure. It is the specific geometric structure of molecular arrangement that determines a crystal's properties, and all crystals are classified by science into seven types of crystals, based on the primary geometric formation in their lattice structure.

Crystals, particularly Quartz crystals, vibrate at such a consistent rate (because of the organization and structural integrity of their molecular structure and arrangement of $SiO_2$) that you can time a watch to it – quite literally. The first, and best, watches are based on a small piece of precisely cut quartz crystal, which generates its own power through the generation of electricity as a result of the mechanical pressure of being 'squeezed', and vibrates consistently to measure the passing of seconds on the watch. Crystals struck underwater, which causes them to vibrate and emit piezoelectricity and electromagnetic frequencies, created the first sonar wave. The first radios were crystal based, and by adjusting the tuning dial on your radio, one could effectively 'tune' the inner quartz crystal to establish resonance with a particular radio station, vibrating on its same frequency and enabling it to receive information, which could then be processed and translated as audible sound. It is thus easy to see how incoherence, or non-coherence, is akin to static on the radio, or an unclear station. It is also easy to see how important resonance is when it comes to information transfer – if the crystal is tuned just a fraction from the precise frequency of the radio signal, there is a dramatic decrease in the amount *and* integrity of the information that can be received, processed, and transmitted. Crystals are so integral to the development of our technological advancements, from radios and satellites to computer processing, because of the perfect and coherent frequencies and patterns that can be achieved by them. As we shall see, it is the perfection, coherence, and structure of these frequencies and patterns that makes crystals unique in their effect on the organization and structure of water.

CHAPTER 7

# THE (CRITICAL) NATURE OF
# PATTERNS

---

*There are only patterns, patterns on top of patterns, patterns
that affect other patterns. Patterns hidden by patterns. Patterns
within patterns. If you watch close, history does nothing but
repeat itself. What we call chaos is just patterns we haven't
recognized. What we call random is just patterns we can't
decipher. What we can't understand we call nonsense. What
we can't read we call gibberish.*
~CHUCK PALAHNIUK
JOURNALIST, NOVELIST

*Nature uses only the longest threads to weave her patterns, so that
each small piece of her fabric reveals the organization of the entire
tapestry.*
~RICHARD FEYNMAN
NOBEL PRIZE, PHYSICS
THE CHARACTER OF PHYSICAL LAW (1965)

Patterns are *everywhere*. All of Nature is based on
geometries, vectors, vertices, patterns, and fractals. From
the macrocosmic to the microcosmic, we see the
intelligence of patterns as the basis of Creation. Our
understanding of our natural environment is dependent

upon us recognizing the patterns that exist in all of the many expressions of nature. Plants grow, branch, and leaf in precise ratios and patterns of development for optimum health. Seashells display exquisite Fibonacci spirals. Coral, sea slugs, and leafy greens display the once theoretical "hyperbolic geometries" – hyperbolic referring to a type of curved space where two parallel lines actually *can* reach the same point. These geometries, which operate in a curved space, were once thought by modern mathematicians to exist only in imaginary, "hyperbolic space". These mathematicians had spent too much time thinking in terms of the traditional flat, 2-dimensional, and completely *un-curved* mythical plane of Euclidean space – the imaginary realm where most mathematics are performed and the flat lines and space we are given to work in when conducting graphs, measurements, examining angles, and even visualizing electromagnetic waves – which of course, cannot be 2-dimensional (as nothing in our Universe is). Had these mathematicians simply paid a little more attention to the patterns they observe in our natural world and life (rather than the patterns and rules they follow in imaginary, 'flat-space'), hyperbolic geometries would have never been theoretical in the first place. Instead, mathematicians would have recognized these geometries amongst ocean life, salad plates, or dried apples, which express these shapes in their normal appearance.[1] Indeed, *learning itself* is based on pattern recognition, which determines everything from the perception of our environment to our awareness of patterns of behavior or situations. Even the visual perception of our surroundings – what we see when we look around us – is largely based upon pattern

---

1. Wertheim, Margaret. "The Beautiful Math of Coral."Presented at the TED2009 Conference, Long Beach, CA, February 2009.

recognition. One experiment demonstrated that kittens, when raised in an environment lacking either horizontal or vertical lines, would *fail to recognize these lines when exposed to an environment containing them.* Kittens raised with only vertical lines could not recognize horizontal lines, and likewise kittens raised with only horizontal lines were unable to recognize and respond to vertical lines. Needless to say, this caused quite a catastrophe when the kittens became exposed to a new environment with these lines and structures they did not perceive. Some cats appear to never be able to recognize these lines again, while other cats seemed to experience a learning curve of recognition, during which time (it is assumed) they recognize the new patterns of experience based on the effect of these new vertical lines in their environment. Their brain and visual perception appears to open to incorporate these new rules of their surroundings – rules that involve the existence of *both* horizontal and vertical lines.[2] This type of work has massive implications for the importance of patterns and our potential ability to only see what we have *learned* to see, akin to a type of developmental visual conditioning. Even *germs* were discovered by the recognition of patterns, when a Hungarian physician recognized the pattern between washed and unwashed hands in regards to the incidence of infections. Although he couldn't offer any scientific explanation for the benefit of hand washing, Dr. Ignaz Semmelweis recognized the pattern of the rise of infant mortality rates and infections when the doctor's hands were not washed, years before the "Germ Theory" was confirmed by Louis Pasteur and others (shortly after Semmelweis's death). Unfortunately, Dr. Semmelweis was not as well received as Pasteur – instead he was

2. Gerber, Richard, M.D. 2001.

ridiculed by the medical community, who denied his desperate insistence they adopt his hand washing methods, and was committed to an insane asylum where he was beaten to death by guards.[3] The story of Semmelweis itself represents a pattern – he is not the first doctor or scientist to be ridiculed, jailed, or committed for their discovery. Medicine, Science, Biology, Physics, and Astronomy are all based on patterns. Even the study of psychology and behavior – any kind of behavior – is completely based on patterns, because our psychology and behavior are pattern based. We make personal judgments, relationship decisions, and our life choices all based on pattern recognition.

> ...but according to patterns, rules, or as we call them, Laws of Nature.
> ~CARL SAGAN

The intelligence of patterns goes far deeper than our astronomical, biological, or psychological patterns. It pervades our existence from the highest levels – the macrocosm of our Universe – down to the microcosmic, the atomic and molecular levels of patterns of geometric structures and organizations. Beyond even than that, the intelligence of patterns reaches into the levels of magnetism and energetics, wherein there exists patterns of geometric structures and organizations, which give rise to the manifestation of energetic fields and their own corresponding geometric patterns and organization – creating the morphogenetic fields in which we operate and the matrix of consciousness in which Creation and

3. Carter, K. Codell and Barbara R. *Childbed Fever: A Scientific Biography of Ignaz Semmelweis, Contributions in Medical Studies.* Westport, CT: Greenwood Press, 1994.

being-ness manifest. Morphogenetic fields (also called morphic or morphogenic fields) are described by Rupert Sheldrake and others as energy fields that constitute a "species specific" Collective Memory, much like the Collective Consciousness described by the great psychologist Carl Jung. This *collective consciousness memory* is information contained in an energetic field, a field that is dynamic and ever changing, constantly storing and updating its information in its patterns. This energetic field contains information to which we have access – access to retrieve information as well as to contribute information. These "morphogenetic fields" are said to account for the information that is critical for an organism to develop from embryo to adult, information and ancestral memory that is not present in our DNA. This information is necessary for our existence, development, and evolution, and the theory developed by Rupert Sheldrake is well-founded in strong support for the existence of such morphogenetic fields, which he defines as: "the organizing fields of animal and human behavior, of social and cultural systems, and of mental activity can all be regarded as morphic fields which contain an inherent memory."[4] (Rupert Sheldrake, *The Presence of the Past*) What he describes are patterns of energy, which contain information. From the smallest seashells to the apparent empty space around us, we are surrounded by patterns. Through our evolution, humans have come to understand that *patterns contain information,* and that by recognizing patterns we can incorporate new information into our understanding and adjust how we interact with our environment for our benefit. Patterns are how we learn, and patterns are the rules of our

4. Sheldrake, Rupert. *The Presence of the Past: Morphic Resonance and the Habits of Nature*. New York, NY: Times Books, 1988, Reprint 1995.

Universe. Recall the importance of the *structure* of the protein molecule, rather than its chemical composition – the pattern of structure carries the information. Electromagnetic and energy waves express this concept very well. We are told that all waves persist or travel in a pattern, which includes its waveform, amplitude, and frequency. This specific pattern of waveform, amplitude, and frequency carries the energetic information, be it sound, light, satellite, cell phone waves, Wi-Fi waves, or human emotional and energetic emissions. At the foundation of our existence, we find that all energy is information, and is encoded in patterns. This holds true whether speaking of the patterns of electromagnetic activity, subtle energy, or the even less tangible patterns of emotional connections and consciousness. These patterns of energy must be processed and translated by our systems in order for us to appropriately respond to the new level of information. This is most easily seen in our sensory perceptions, where patterns of energy – whether audible sound, visual light, patterns of aroma, etc. – are processed by our systems into understandable information that we then use to establish a functioning perception of our environment and existence. In reality, our bodies, through our senses, are providing us our experience of our physical reality only by recognizing and interacting with patterns. The reality of our physical experience and the fundamental mechanics of our electromagnetic universe dictate an extremely interesting reality, as discussed by physicists like Michio Kaku and others, in that *nothing* in our Universe actually comes into contact with anything else. Because there is a space surrounding all atoms, which consist of a strong electromagnetic field where electrons – particles of charged energy – are bouncing, zipping, and moving around, it is not the actual *atom* that comes into contact with other atoms, instead it is only the electromagnetic fields that are touching and interacting. We don't actually touch anything – rather, the extremely dense electromagnetic energy of our body, which carries and conducts information, comes into contact with the extremely dense electromagnetic energy of the thing we are touching. The *patterns* of electromagnetic energy of the thing we are touching are the only things with which we are truly interacting, and *our* electromagnetic fields in turn decode these patterns into information which it can then process as sensory information. Even when you *feel* as though you are touching something, it is really nerves zipping up electricity through your body in decodable patterns for processing in the brain. It is the *pattern of energy* that tell us whether a thing is soft or hard, fuzzy or smooth, sweet or salty. The same applies to sound and light, which are more obvious examples of this principle. Light waves (a.k.a. electromagnetic energy waves) are received by the electromagnetic energy fields of our eyes, which translates the patterns of light into information processed by the brain to relay a certain color, shade, or otherwise visual perception. Sound waves (a.k.a. patterned electromagnetic energy waves) reach the electromagnetic fields of our eardrums and canals, where the patterns of the waves are decoded into audible sound. In essence, it is truly the crystallographic patterned nature of our energetic and electromagnetic Universe, interacting with the liquid crystallographic patterned nature of our physical system, which allows us to experience the sensations of this amazing existence. Patterns interacting with patterns, and patterned energetic fields interacting with and in water. There are many other patterns of energy and information outside of our perceivable senses of touch, sound, taste, smell, and sight. There are so many other patterns of energy and information in fact, that on a spectrum chart of the known different electromagnetic energy patterns, those that are perceivable to our senses represent an *extremely* small and *very* insignificant percentage. While we may not be able to *perceive* these different electromagnetic frequencies, we are still responding to them nearly every moment, whether we are consciously aware of it or not. These different frequency patterns have been shown to have *enormous* impacts on Life and human health. In addition to electromagnetic frequency patterns, there are also patterns of subtle energy and *magneto-electricity* – energies that may not be detectable but for which there is substantial support for their existence and actions. All of these energies are abundant in our environment and are proven to have marked effects on our minds, bodies, and spirits. And there are the patterns of consciousness; the intangible patterns of experience, thought, and behavior, which we now know have power well beyond that which science has acknowledged. Our patterns of consciousness are the major driving force of our wellness, and they can have immediate and dramatic effects on our minds, bodies, and spirits. The evidence for this lies in every motivating lecture, effective psychological therapy, and every consciousness-based healing and miracle experienced throughout time, from the ancient faith healings of our world's religions to the modern day effective psychological therapies, energy healing practices, and the everyday healing miracles of the effect of consciousness, including events such as the witnessed and documented dissipating cancer tumors during the chants of a group of monks. Such an event cannot be reduced to the effect of the sound created by such chanting, it is the result of a consciousness-based energetic effect – which, like everything else, operates on patterns. Our body receives all of these patterns of energy, whether that information is translated by our sensory perceptions or not. Not only are our audio and visual range a very small portion of the electromagnetic scale, they also operates within a filter system in the brain, which only processes in our conscious mind a *very* small percentage of the information it actually receives as useable. It is theorized that the *massive* amount of information that does not get consciously processed is still stored somewhere within the body or mind – that intangible place of subconscious and conscious memory storage, which exists within the structure of our water system rather than a localized section of the brain or body, as we will soon discuss. We know that all kinds of energy affect our systems, and thus we know that our bodies are receiving and reacting to incoming energy and information of which we are unaware. But *how* is our body able to perform such amazing feats, on a *constant* basis? How can it possibly be receiving so much information, akin to an incredibly dynamic antenna, and how can it possibly process and react to so much information, more complex than the most advanced computing system we could ever dream of? It does so through our water system, which acts as an antenna and interface between energy and our physical systems, and between information and our experience. We already know that water has a profound responsiveness to consciousness, subtle energy, and magnetism, as well as electromagnetic information. Water reacts to the patterns of information to which it is exposed – whether consciousness and subtle energy or electromagnetic information – and rearranges its own pattern (or structure) accordingly to incorporate the new information. This phenomenon also occurs in the water in our bodies, where new information is expressed as a change in pattern and has the largest impact on our energetic and physical systems, a phenomena we will examine when discussing our body's water system and the physical and energetic interface properties of our bio-waters.

*Information in the form of Energy, streams in simultaneously through all of our sensory systems. And then it explodes into this enormous collage of what this present moment looks like, what it feels like, and what it sounds like.*
~ DR. JILL BOLTE TAYLOR
NEUROSCIENTIST

# CHAPTER 8

# ENERGY, ENTROPY, AND GEOMETRY

---

Because energy is always information, and information persists and is encoded in patterns, we can thus understand that *energy exists within patterns*. In the world of pattern, structure, and energy, we encounter two different forces, or polarities. One is *entropy*, or *entropic structures*, while the other is *non-entropy*, *non-entropic structures*, *or syntropic structures*.

The term *entropy* has more than one definition within physics, and these definitions have changed more than once. Here, we use the term *entropy* in its reference to the process of something that, left alone over time, will gradually decline into disorder, i.e. the process of life and death. All organic-based systems and materials experience a level of entropy, and will decay over time. Negative entropy, also termed 'syntropy', refers to the opposite occurrence – something which does not decay or decline, but instead when left alone over time will progress or change into a state of higher function and order, and is presumed to be theoretical. Classical physics also teaches that everything except a (theoretical) perfect crystal experiences entropy, while the (theoretical) perfect crystal experiences "zero entropy" (Newton's

Third Law of Thermodynamics), because of the *perfect precision* of the crystal's geometrically arranged atomic and molecular structural form. The perfect structure of this perfect crystal would maintain its structural integrity despite the forces of nature, such as gravity compression, which over time would cause decay in an imperfect structure. Thus, crystalline structures, because of their mathematically precise, highly ordered, geometrically arranged lattice structures, are held to represent the lowest entropic state possible.

Here we understand that *precise geometric structures* can allow crystals to persist without decay, and that precise geometric structures are the best patterns and forms to contain the largest amount of sustainable information, information that can persist because it is not contained in a more entropic structure, which over time experiences *loss of information* in its decay process. A solid-state crystal, because of the precise structure of lines and angles (also called *vectors* and *vertices*) within its molecular organization and structure, represents our highest potential for information storage and retrieval. This is because the angles, vertices, or points of intersection within its structure are in precise mathematical relationships – the same reason why it represents the lowest entropic state possible. The precise angles of these *vertices* or points of intersection allow for the high structural integrity, which translates into the lowest entropy, or susceptibility for decay, possible. It is for this reason that the quartz hard drives developed by Hitachi are said to last for millions of years and still hold their data – data which is encoded into these vertices using lasers.

Since water is a flexible and responsive liquid crystal, it can exhibit an infinite combination of patterns, vectors, vertices, and geometries within its remarkably small molecular arrangement. Some patterns, such as those found in the waters of municipal systems, polluted environments, waters exposed to harmful and artificial electromagnetic frequencies, or even waters treated by severely depressed patients as witnessed by Grad during his experiments, are highly entropic. They lack the symmetry and organization of geometric arrangements that provide structural integrity, and without this they are on a rapid path of decay and decline. The more highly structured the water is, the more organized and complex crystallographic patterns it holds, the more non-entropic its geometric structural integrity – whether structured through light, sound, frequency, movement, or natural location (i.e. certain glacial waters or healing water sources such as the Lourdes). When it comes to the water in our body, the more non-entropic and highly structured it is, the more energy it contains, the more information it holds, and the longer it maintains its ability to support our physical and energetic systems – including the integrity of our DNA.

# CHAPTER 9

# A WORD ON FRACTALS

The term *fractal* might seem a bit daunting at first, but the concept is actually a very easy to grasp, and an important one that you will begin to see in all of Nature once you understand it. *Fractals* are found in the roughness in Nature – the jagged lines and unsmooth edges that at first appear random, but when studied under microscopes display amazing mathematical relationships and patterns. It is a shape that can be split into parts, usually under greater and greater magnification, where we see that each part is (approximately) a reduced-size copy of the whole – a property called "self-similarity." Fractals are the beautiful symmetry of self-repeating and self-similar patterns that we see in plants, coral, and snowflakes. The concept of fractals involves the angles and edges of things, its complex patterns, and the "as above, so below" axiom principle. Investigating the wonder of fractals is the only way to grasp the capacity for immense information storage, the complexity of the patterns on which our existence is based, and to gain a context of what the intense complexity of pattern potential within our water means for our DNA and physical and bio-energetic systems. In order to truly recognize Water, we must acknowledge Water's, and Nature's, fractality. The fractality of our Universe, and indeed the whole concept of fractals, is important when conceptualizing how structured Water operates as a fractal antenna – one of its most fundamental properties.

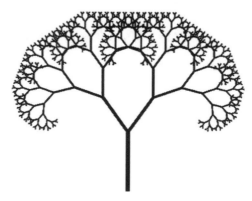

Fig. 10: Fractal tree pattern. Note repeating similar pattern on smaller scales.

*Fractals,* and more specifically, *fractal geometry,* is the name coined by mathematician Benoit Mandelbrot in 1975 to describe repeating or self-similar mathematical patterns. Derived from the Latin *fractus,* meaning "broken" or "fractured", fractal patterns have been found in sound, nature, technology, art, and even law. Although these repeating and self-similar patterns are viewable everywhere in Nature, this form of geometry was previously unidentified by the scientific community. Mandelbrot was the first to discover the mathematical algorithms to produce fractal geometries, and the first to chart these principles within the parameters of mathematics in the modern scientific world. Like Dr. Marcel Vogel, Benoit Mandelbrot was also an IBM researcher, and the story surrounding his discovery of fractal geometry and patterns helps express its concepts. Recruited by IBM to help solve the problem of a natural white noise interference that was interrupting the transfer of computer data over phone lines, Mandelbrot applied his natural technique of thinking visually (rather than analytically) to the issue. He "instinctually looked at the white noise in terms of the shapes it generated – an early form of IBM's now-renowned data visualization practices...Regardless of the scale of the graph, whether it represented data over the course of one day, one hour, or one second, the pattern...was surprisingly familiar. There was a larger structure at work."[1] This observation led to his mathematical calculations of *fractal geometries*, which express these smaller sub-units of similar patterns, and caused a breakthrough in modern science.

*In the whole of science, the whole of mathematics, smoothness was everything. What I did was to open up roughness for investigation.*
~BENOIT MANDELBROT
MATHEMATICIAN

Modern science, mathematics, medicine, education, and society are built on the concept of *measurement*, which requires smoothness. But the truth of the matter is that nothing in Nature is completely smooth, and nothing in Nature can be measured. Stephen Harrod Buhner beautifully explains this phenomenon, eloquently describing that when it comes to actually *measuring a line in Nature*, it cannot truly be done. We try, and give sufficient approximations, but every time we look closer at an object in Nature, when we view it under stronger magnification, we find that the line becomes more jagged

1. *IBM Icons of Progress: Fractal Geometry.* IBM. Web. 23 Dec 2013.

and irregular. To truly measure the object, each one of the lines and angles would have to be measured as well. And each time we zoom in closer, we see even more angles and jagged edges. Think of this through practical application – it is impossible, for example, to accurately measure the circumference of a tree. When we calculate this with a tape measure, we are eliminating all of the curves and angles in the bark of a tree. If an ant were to walk the circumference of that tree, he would be crossing hills and valleys along his way, adding significantly to the distance traveled. If something even smaller than the ant were to journey the circumference of the tree, what were hills and valleys to the ant suddenly become mountains and deep gorges, rocky and uneven terrain. If you were to segment out a portion of the bark of the tree, or any line in Nature for that matter, and magnify it, you will find it is even more wrinkled, irregular, and jagged than you could see with just your eyes, and that these wrinkled, irregular, and jagged lines follow the same pattern as those we saw before it was magnified. If you segment out of a portion of *that* line, and magnify it even more, you will see the same, and so on and so forth, all following similar to the original pattern of irregular wrinkled lines we saw in the first place. To *truly* measure these lines, we would find ourselves getting to continuously and continuously smaller units of scale, until we are no longer able to magnify because of technological limits, or until the lines between matter and non-matter begin to dissipate, as we see when we reach into the atomic structure of particles and find ourselves in the realm of quantum physics, where atoms and space do not seem to "obey the rules". This is a most basic concept of fractals – a patterns that expresses smaller and smaller similar patterns as it is examined more closely, and the jagged lines and edges of things which express information.

And so it is with Nature. In all of Nature, you will never find a straight line. Upon closer observation, you will find that every line is wrinkled, irregular, and jagged, when viewed from any perspective. This is the pattern of our Universe, the *non-linear* nature of Nature, demonstrating its capacity for infinity simply by being impossible to measure. When modern science, mathematics, medicine, education, and society is built on the concept of *measurement,* and nothing in Nature can truly be measured, it is no surprise we find ourselves at odds with our environment, living in a realm of attempting to control it while never understanding it. A popular psychological researcher described a professor as teaching "If it can't be measured, it doesn't exist." Actually, it is the other way around – the concept of *measurement* only exists in imaginary, 2-dimensional flat imaginary Euclidean space, where everything is completely smooth and space is completely uncurved. The space in our Universe, and of our Earth, is most certainly curved, as postulated by Einstein (and later proved), and nothing is ever truly smooth. The reality is if it *can* be measured, it doesn't exist. Nothing in Nature can be Measured – for it is All based on Fractality – similar patterns that continue on in smaller and smaller units of scale.

> *Thus a fractal... is a nonlinear object composed of subunits (and sub-sub-units) that resemble the larger structure. All fractal objects possess this property, known as self-similarity; while they are highly irregular, they also have patterns... this also applies to any processes or properties the objects may have, such as velocity, pressure, and*

*temperature. Every property of a natural object will,*
*when examined, display a fractal nature.*
~STEPHEN HARROD BUHNER

The important thing to remember about the fractality
of nature, and thus the fractality of water, geometry, and
our physical systems and processes, is that *fractals allow*
*for infinite potentials of information.* Let's talk about how
this works. Take an electromagnetic wave, for example.
Electromagnetic waves are much more complex than the
simple line figures typically associated with them. Like
everything else in Nature, electromagnetic waves are
fractals. Their vibrations are not merely the amplitude,
modulation, and the frequency; they are also the
reverberations *within* the wave pattern. Here, we mean
the "waves within the waves". Because there are no
straight lines, as we zoom in closer and closer to the
wave pattern we see that it, too, is jagged and wavy – i.e.
fractalized. Stephen Harrod Buhner, renowned author,
lecturer, and senior researcher for the Foundation for
Gaian Studies, eloquently describes the fractality of
electromagnetic waves, also called "sine waves" in
mathematics, which express a repetitive and curving
pattern. In one of his books, *The Secret Teachings of Plants*,
he states,

> *Electromagnetic spectrum signals, like those we*
> *know as a particular radio station, can and do*
> *contain very large amounts of information...* And
> when life flows through the electromagnetic
> spectrum, when it flows through a particular
> frequency, it fractalizes it, just as other
> dimensional lines fractalize. The oscillating sine
> wave or broadband frequency that life flows

through becomes a fractal and its edges take on the same kind of irregular shaping that solid objects do. Every time life flows through a frequency on the electromagnetic spectrum, it fractalizes that wave differently, because the flow of life is always nonlinear. What is interesting is that unique information is always embedded or encoded within the way the oscillating sine wave is fractalized... *Radio waves carry information in much the same way. A pure oscillating sine wave of a particular frequency is created and that wave is disturbed, the smoothness of its line fractured, by the particular kinds of information that the radio station puts into it.* (Waves on the ocean are a visual example of oscillatory fractalized sine waves. They move up and down – oscillate – and their surfaces are rough – fractalized.)[2] (emphasis added)

These electromagnetic waves do not exist in imaginary, 2-dimensional Euclidean space, flat objects on a flat background, as commonly depicted by the machines we developed to detect them and our classic textbooks. Rather, electromagnetic waves travel, propagate, or at the very least exist, within the multi-dimensional Universe. As Nassim Haramein so eloquently points out in his lecture *The Event Horizon*, electromagnetic waves are (at least) 3-dimensional, and would thus actually appear as a spiral throughout or within space, rather than function as a theoretical 2-dimensional line.

Electromagnetic waves are not only fractalized, containing immense amounts of information within their

---

2. Buhner, Stephen Harrod. *Secret Teaching of Plants.* Rochester, Vermont: Bear and Co., 2004.

irregular faceting and fractal lines, they are fractalized within *at least* 3 dimensions, making this irregularity and fractality even more intricate and complex than previously imagined, and allowing for an even greater encoding of information. These fractal lines, these irregularities and wrinkles on and within the wave, which contain sub-units along their lines of even more wrinkled lines, sub-sub-sub units that are assumed to continue on into infinity – these fractal lines are creating complex, geometric, and precise patterns of information within their seemingly irregular, non-linear nature. Thus we can then expand our visual representation of electromagnetic waves from their flat, 2-dimensional textbook depictions to a more realistic view of spiraling, vortices of energy, of infinitely complex fractals, containing potentially infinite amounts of information. *Electromagnetic energy waves are actually patterns in motion – complex geometric patterns of infinite information.*

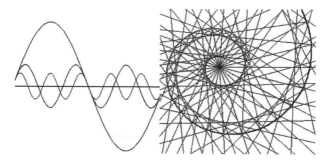

Fig. 11: Classic textbook depiction of
electromagnetic waves (left) vs. Fractalized
spiraling vortex wave (right).

Radio waves are not the only fractal patterns in motion. All energy, all forms, and indeed our entire Universe, is comprised of fractal patterns in motion. According to IBM, "Fractal patterns have appeared in almost all of the physiological processes within our bodies. For ages, the human heart was believed to beat in a regular, linear fashion, but recent studies have shown that the true rhythm of a healthy heart fluctuates radically in a distinctively fractal pattern. Blood is also distributed throughout the body in a fractal manner. Researchers in Toronto are using ultrasound imaging to identify the fractal characteristics of blood flows in both healthy and diseased kidneys...the hope is to measure the fractal dimensions of these blood flows, and use mathematical models to detect cancerous cell formations sooner than ever before..."[3]

More than just our physiology, fractals have impacted nearly every field of development. Graphic design and image editing software now use fractals to create incredibly life-like special effects, and beautiful, complex, and more natural looking landscapes. How much carbon dioxide the world can safely process can be measured, or at least quantified, by applying fractal statistical analyses to forests. Weather patterns, galaxy clusters, formations and organisms, and even stock market price variations, have all proven to be fractal in nature.[4]

Fractal antennas were the saving grace development that allowed for the explosion in cellphones and hand held devices, making possible all of today's smartphones, Wi-Fi, and GPS capabilities. Most people have no idea that their cellular phone is likely equipped with a fractal antenna, which it uses to receive and transmit large amounts of information. These antennas do not look like the long extension rod from our original cell phones and

3. IBM. "Icons of Progress: Fractal Geometry."
4. IBM. "Icons of Progress: Fractal Geometry."

cordless phones, rather the antenna is folded in upon
itself in repeating patterns and looks more like a
snowflake, thus fitting into a smaller space and using
several geometrically precise angles and vertices to
receive and transmit information. Fractalizing the
antenna, i.e. creating similar smaller repeating patterns,
also called self-similar sub-units (and sub-sub-units –
essentially folding the common antenna upon itself) –
on geometric patterns and specific guidelines, increases
the amount of material or surface area that can send and
receive information. This allows for a massive expansion
of the "receivable and transmissible bandwidth" –
meaning that the cellular phone, for example, can now
send and receive at lower frequencies and at higher
frequencies than it could before.

The *frequency bandwidth* refers to the range of
electromagnetic frequencies on which a device operates
to send and receive information. For example, the
frequency bandwidth of a specific radio station might be
91.3 FM, where the FM stands for Frequency Modulation
(number of cycles, or repetitions, per second), and the AM
stands for Amplitude Modulation (the size of the pattern,
rather than its number of repetitions). In radio, the FM
dial creates different frequencies, or electromagnetic
waves, by changing the number of cycles, or repetitions,
the wave repeats itself each second. Each radio station
on the FM dial has a slightly different pattern of cycles
per second. On the AM dial of your radio station, the
electromagnetic waves are differentiated for different
radio stations by adjusting the amplitude, or size of the
wave (as in the height of its peak on the wave) and not
its number of cycles per second. Every individual radio
station now has their own specific electromagnetic

bandwidth wave they can now fractalize with the information of their specific station.

The frequency bandwidth of cellular phones used to be in the 100-300 MHz range (100-300 millions of cycles per second). However, with the rapid and continuous growth of the technological era and its advancements and the astronomical rise in cellular phone style communications, the frequency bandwidth of cellular phones has risen past 3 GHz, meaning the frequencies are operating at a speed of 3 *billion* cycles per second, simply to allow for the massive number of them in use. All of these frequency band expansions create a ton of interference, and the air around us is not as invisible as it appears. Cellphone signals, Wi-Fi signals, radio waves, and other sources of electromagnetic frequencies are all occupying our airwaves, and potentially interfere with each other, making signals slow, interrupted, and weak. Most of our cellphones and Wi-Fi routers would not be able to operate well under such conditions as the polluted airwaves of today, and would certainly not be able to send and receive GPS signals or Wi-Fi information, if not for the recent development of the fractal antenna, which also allows for the expansion in bandwidth (or the frequency speed at which information can be received and transmitted). Without the development of the fractal antenna, our cellphones and Wi-Fi routers probably wouldn't be able to operate, or at the very least would have even longer and bulkier antennas than they used to. The fractal antenna, which looks more like a snowflake than a our traditional image of an "antenna", allows for a greater surface area of information transmission as well as greater storage and processing capabilities, because the information it receives and transmits is more *coherent* thanks to the nature of fractal antennas. Information stored and transmitted along fractal patterns is more organized, making the information more synchronized and coherent so that it can be processed *without* experiencing a great loss of information (which occurs in incoherent information transfer, where large amounts of information becomes unorganized and therefore becomes essentially nonsense, the full amount of information unable to be processed and thus lost). To allow for such massive amounts of information and transfer capacity in such a small space as our smartphones, the fractality of the antenna allows the system to transfer massive amounts of data in an incredibly small system.

The fractality of water, which also serves as an antenna – receiving and transferring information – allows water the same capacity as the fractal antennas in our cellular phones, transferring vast amounts of information in an incredibly small space. This concept is not so different from the holographic theory, which could only be possible through the fractality of structure. The holographic theory proposes that our Universe is much like a hologram, because each piece of a hologram contains all of the information of the whole. In this context, each piece of the Universe contains *all* of the information of the entire cosmos and conscious Universe – something that would only be possible through the nature of fractality, where massive amounts of information can be received, stored, and transferred in the smallest of spaces due to the complex self-similar sub-units of angles and geometric patterns. These angles, vertices, and geometric patterns are responsible not only for storing information, but also to allow for its coherent reception and transmission. The only possible way that each piece of the Universe could contain *all of the*

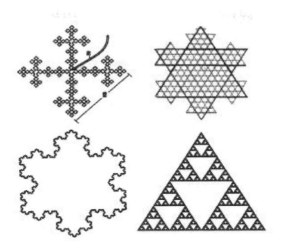

Fig. 12: Examples of fractal antennas.
Notice the similarity to snowflakes, as well as
the resemblance to honored and revered
shapes and images, including the Star of
David (top right).
Images: Top left: Nathan Cohen, "Fractal
antennas and fractal resonators" U.S. Patent
6,452,553. Remaining Images: Yale
University, classes.yale.edu/fractals

*information of the whole* is through the fractal nature of
Nature.

Thus we arrive at the beautiful nature of Water's
properties as a fractal antenna. The structure of Water,
like everything else in Nature, is of course fractal. We can
see this in the beautiful snowflake ice crystals we are all
familiar with. Thanks to the work of researchers like Dr.
Masaru Emoto and Prof. Korotkov, we are also able to
view the expression of Water's fractal patterns and how
they relate to its stored energetic information. It would
appear that the greater the Life-supporting energy and

information stored in the water's structure, the greater the display of fractal form. Conversely, the more damaging, or non-Life-supporting, energy and information stored in its structure, the greater the display of *loss* of fractality and form. The water in our bodies, and in fact the bio-water in *all* living things and self-organized systems, is highly structured and fractal. In fact, Water's functions as a Life-supporting element are dependent upon this structure. This alone is a revolutionary understanding, as it implies that it is not necessarily *Water* that is necessary for Life, it is *Structured Liquid Crystalline Water.* And we are full of it – responsive, interactive, and dynamic liquid crystal Water, called the world's most malleable computer, equipped with the most complex fractal antenna network system imaginable.

Let's take a moment to explore this complexity, as it helps to realize the great power and potentials of 99.95% of your molecules. Water is able to receive and transmit *mass* amounts of information and energy via its molecular arrangement of complex fractal patterns within its bond arrangements. Each sub-unit, each line, and each segment of line, as well its angles and vertices, or points of intersections, transmit, receive, and contain information. Recall that each memory cell unit of water is comprised of an average of 3 to 60 water molecules grouped together, and can contain at least 440,000 panels of information. Here, we should recognize that these are fractal panels for information storage within the angles and vertices of its structure, and the number represented is likely the smallest sub-unit perceived specifically for this observation or study. Since greater magnification would reveal greater fractality and thus more panels for information storage, 440,000 panels per water cell unit becomes a very conservative estimate. When we consider that the human body potentially contains **one million trillion trillion molecules, 99.9% of which are water,** we realize that the amount of information stored within the fractal pattern of our water is *incalculable,* as is the amount of information we, as water-based individuals, are capable of receiving and transmitting. Thus how we view of our bodies begins to undergo a massive shift towards a much more accurate representation of our physical systems, as a dynamic, water-based, fractal antenna.

CHAPTER 10

# EVERYTHING IS CRYSTALLOGRAPHY

---

*The stellar universe ought to be a finite island in the infinite ocean (crucible) of space.*
~EINSTEIN

As science continues to explore deeper down the rabbit hole of our manifested reality, it continues to convey an ultimate truth regarding the fundamentals of our physical universe and the forces of energy driving it – that in fact, *everything is crystallography.* Thus new research has begun into the growing understanding of *structured energy,* where science recognizes that all energies, whether they are seen, unseen, magnetic fields, or even consciousness based, operate on principles of pattern and structure. Through this realization, we begin to glimpse behind the veil of our physical constructs into the realm of the energetic template which gives rise to all that is manifest. As the structure of water is so intimately connected with the structure of consciousness and energy, it is prudent here to apply what we have learned regarding the mechanisms and principles surrounding structured water to the mechanisms and principles surrounding the structure of energy.

It has been proposed by many physicists and scientists that not only do we exist in a dynamic sea of energy, invisible to our extremely limited ability to perceive electromagnetic frequencies, but that there is also a definite *structure* to the energy around us. The structure of the energy of an environment provides us with information and interacts with the energy of ourselves. One of the vital functions of our electromagnetic fields is to interpret and react to information that it encounters. The structure of the energy around us is what we are reacting to when we experience a sense of peace in one area, or feel the tension that can be "cut with a knife" in another. It is the unseen fluid and changeable geometrical pattern of the matrix of an environment, upon which information travels nearly instantly. It is the operating principle behind the development of theories such as dark matter or morphogenic fields, it is the mechanism by which healing prayer, distance healing, and out of body experiences occur, and it is the quality that the principles of Feng Shui are influencing and adapting in its application. It is the geometrical "structure of the vacuum" that physicist Nassim Haramein describes in his work, and the Field that Einstein described when he spoke of "the field" being the "sole governing force of the particle."

The topic of structured energy answers the currently unexplainable way that light acts in our Universe and our bodies, how birds and other animals communicate with each other instantly, how eggs form living beings, and how healing energies and other energies move at faster than light speed. When one understands that there is a *structure* to the energy in our Universe, and that this structure is *highly changeable and influenceable,* much like the structure of liquid crystal Water, there is a greater understanding of one's relationship to the structure of energy, how this affects your experience of life, your relationships with all things, and your relationship with our environment. It also teaches you how to create the structure around you and in your environment to better nourish your energetic body and empower the law of attraction in your life.

Throughout antiquity, there has been a pervasive acknowledgement among people of all cultures that man and the cosmos are "interconnected by a ubiquitous, all-pervasive sea of energy that undergirds, and is manifest in, all phenomena."[1] It has been given different names by the various traditions that have discussed it, and has often been called ether, Prana, Qi, and Chi in more ancient traditions, or zero-point energy, dark matter, morphogenetic fields, the consciousness grid, and aether by more modern science groups and Unified Field theories. But all traditions are incomplete or inaccurate in their understanding and description. Perhaps some of the more ancient traditions had a more complete understanding in their antiquity, but it would appear that much knowledge has been lost through changes in civilizations, mistranslations, and evolutions of language. The Reductionist approach that modern man has taken towards our Universe, and the simplification and mechanization of complex non-linear processes, such as that of the heart, brain, and human body, has also played

1. Puthoff, H.E., Ph.D. Physics and Metaphysics as Co-Emergent Phenomena. *Research News and Opportunities in Science and Theology* 2, No. 8, p. 22. Institute of Advanced Studies, Austin: Templeton Foundation Press, April 2002.

a large role in today's misunderstanding of the fundamental structure of energy and our universe.

While often used when describing the spiritual energetics of our Universe, Prana, Chi, and other such terms for the *nutritive life force energy* do not, as far as Western translations are concerned, correctly correspond to the structure of our Universe. These terms deal with another topic altogether, which is the energy of *the vital force of life*, and the spiritual, energetic nutritive substance that pervades all *living* things on our planet. This is the energy force and nutritive substance which flows within our meridians and the energetic channels within our bodies much like blood flows within our veins and is part of our bio-energetic system, which we will explore further in later chapters. The "ether" of Eastern traditions also does not accurately describe the energetics of our Universe, as it classically relates to what Eastern Philosophy calls the "highest" of the five elements of energy of which our Universe is composed (the other four being air, earth, fire, and water). Eastern traditions do come closer to a more accurate definition by describing Ether as 'the essence of emptiness', and the space that all of the other elements fill, but this also is incomplete and inaccurate. The word "aether", coined by early physicists and adopted because of its similarity to the Eastern "ether", has a closer relation to structured energy. Aether was defined by Einstein and others as the medium which fills all space and supports the propagation of electromagnetic waves, although here we also encounter different definitions that refer to aether as being "subtler than light" and being "incapable of change", which is not characteristic of the structure of our Universe. Rather, a more accurate analysis would be "the medium occupying every point in space, including material bodies, and having properties that give rise to the electric and magnetic phenomena, determining the propagation velocity of their effects by the physical properties of the 'aether' or the 'structure of the background energy'". In other words, a definition of "aether" that describes it as the pervasive medium of all space, which has physical qualities that allow for electric and magnetic energy to take place within its medium, and the physical qualities of which determine the rate at which electric and magnetic energies exist within its medium, comes much closer to describing *the structure of the energy of our Universe* – which can be thought of as a type of cosmic microwave background, a dynamic and responsive template of patterns on which the threads of Creation and physical reality are woven and spun.

While there have been extensive experiments done by several great scientists all implying that aether exists, conventional modern science claims to have abandoned the concept of aether and have adopted the term 'zero-point energy' in its stead, which provides them the same basic principles as aether but without having to retract their previous and rather adamant abandonment of it. While Einstein's Theory of Relativity is what originally appeared to have exited aether from physics equations, there is no actual disparity between Einstein's theories and the existence of aether. Einstein himself said that "to deny Aether is ultimately to assume that empty space has no physical qualities whatsoever. The fundamental facts of mechanics do not harmonize with this view."[2] His statement rather clearly states that there is an undeniable background energy and structure to empty space, and thus all space, which has physical qualities.

---

2. Einstein, Albert. "Aether and the Theory of Relativity." Presented at the University of Leyden, Germany, May 5 1920.

It is an important fact that Einstein noted there are
*physical qualities* to the structure of our Universe. This
is *fundamental,* as many conventional physicists prefer to
maintain space as being devoid of physical attributes in
order to make for easier and more simplified equations.
However, the fact remains that *the structure of our Universe,*
even that which we term "empty space", *has definite
physical qualities.* These physical qualities govern the
energy dynamics that take place within its structure, and
determine the electromagnetic waves that are generated
and propagated within their fields. Many great physicists
and scientists, most notably Walter Russell (who was
called the "Leonardo da Vinci of our time" by Walter
Cronkite), have also proposed and demonstrated that
waves do not, in fact, *travel* through space but are
reproduced, or replicated, from "wave-field" to "wave-
field" of space. In this context, a wave-field is the section
of space in which we view an electromagnetic wave in
its full expression of both wavelength and amplitude,
experiencing the full segment of the frequency
information or pattern of the wave in its segmented
entirety – i.e. one full cycle. In his work *The Secret of
Light,* Russell describes how the boundaries of all wave
fields act as mirrors to reflect the light wave from one
field into another, advancing it throughout space/time.
The so-called mirrors, reflecting and refracting the light
wave along its progression from wave-field to wave-field,
*do so because of the geometrical pattern of the structure of the
field.*

> *It will amaze the world to know that those <u>shapes
> of crystals are determined in space by the shapes of
> the wave fields</u> which bound the various elemental
> structures. (emphasis added)*

~WALTER RUSSELL
    PROFESSOR, UNIVERSITY OF SCIENCE AND
    PHILOSOPHY
    THE SECRET OF LIGHT, 1947


Whether termed aether, Chi, Prana, zero-point energy, dark energy, morphogenic fields, the unified field, the consciousness field, or any other name, the basic underlying concept of an all-pervasive field of energy on our planet and within our Universe which allows energetic interactions to take place is a fundamental understanding across all cultures and sciences, and yet each label and associated definitions are incomplete. When it is understood that there is a *structure to energy and a structure to our Universe,* which operates on the same principles of structured water in terms of its responsive, dynamic, and ever-changing nature, we will then be able understand most of our current 'mysteries' – including how information 'travels' and waves are reflected, refracted, or otherwise manifested through space, how our DNA, Nature, and morphogenetic fields are created and applied, the unexplainable intelligence of embryonic development, how consciousness can affect energy patterns, the law of attraction, levitation and anti-gravity, extra-sensory perception, concepts of 'fate' or 'destiny', and how distant and instant healings take place. Understanding the *structure of the Universe* will also help us understand the mechanics of the power of prayer, how energies can move at faster than light speeds, and how to apply this knowledge to better structure the energy of ourselves and our environment, to greater benefit from more highly structured body energetics and water – thus raising our state of wellness and function, structuring the many liquid crystals of the body and brain and the energetic crystal patterns of our electromagnetic and energetic systems. It will also help us to better protect ourselves from the *de-structuring* nature of the energetic contaminants that are polluting the environments around us at magnitudes never before experienced by modern man.

> *In the wave lies the secret of Creation... to know the mechanics of the wave is to know the entire secret of Nature.*
> ~WALTER RUSSELL

The structure of our Universe is a *dynamic crystalline matrix of geometrical patterns,* which directs energy and electromagnetic waves through its field, giving rise to the *qualities* of the waves and energy through their multi-dimensional nature and by methods of refraction and reflection, i.e. the way it moves, bounces, channels, and reflects energy along its template. It is the Matrix of Creation, upon which the Electro-Magnetic Web of Created Physical Reality is woven. It is the means by which the Energy of Source expresses the template of manifestation, the medium through which consciousness causes Creation, a sea of infinite potential void of limitation. It is flexible and dynamic, instantly responsive and subject to subtle changes in consciousness, made of sacred geometrical patterns, and encodes the energy it conducts with the information of its structuring.

Understanding our Universe and environment as being *structured space* explains such things as the intelligence behind the form of development in Nature, the miraculous abilities of the heart's energetic field, and how crystals, plants, and other objects can provide energy to a room or to a person by merely being in its proximity.

It is the *structured environment* that directs where and how energy is transmitted and the information it will carry. Plants, crystals, and other objects placed in a room are contributing to the *structure of the energy within your environment,* creating specific geometrical patterns through which light and localized energy are manifested and transferred, encoding it with the information of the structuring – *thus structuring your energy and the energy being created around you.* This is what truly creates what we term 'ambiance', or the energy and 'feel' of a room. The structured energy of that environment interacts with our structure in a type of energetic dialogue, causing changes in our energy, mood, thought patterns, and our physical bodies, as our own energy fields and water are restructuring to encode the new information of this experience.

The research being done on the structure of water and liquid crystals gives us much insight into how consciousness and other energies affect crystalline geometrical patterns. Images from water that has been exposed to different thoughts, intentions, energies, and environments vary greatly in their expression of structure. These liquid crystal waters are merely expressing the fields created around them. The same is true for the crystalline matrix of our Universe. It has geometrical structure that is similar to but much more dynamic and dimensional than that of water, and also reforms itself instantly when encountering different forms of consciousness or energy. If one were able to observe the different geometrical patterns of the structure of our Universe, one would see how different frequencies and emanations from solar and planetary bodies affect the geometrical patterns of the structure around them, and project this structuring throughout the

cosmos. One would also see the dynamic patterns created
when energies combine and interact with each other
within space. In our own environment, we would be able
to see how different objects, frequencies, and conscious
thought contribute to the complexity or simplification
of the structure of the field around us, and make
correlations between the level of entropy of the structure
and what manifests in reality as a result. Generally
speaking and confirmed through experiments done with
structured water, energies of the highest and most life-
contributing sources form complex geometries, while
energies of a negative or harmful source create more
simplified, distorted, and non-geometric shapes.

In previous stages of our existence we lived in more
pristine environments, structured with the consciousness
and life on and in the Earth, patterning that was further
structured by the patterns of the cosmos. Today, we live in
a world saturated and bombarded with pollutants. They
have contaminated every aspect of our environment –
our food, our air, our land, our space, and our energy.
From toxic chemicals to harmful electromagnetic
frequencies (EMF's), the energetics of our environment
is being *de-structured* at an astronomical and exponential
rate. The implications of this are incalculable. As the
structural integrity of the matrix of our environmental
field is degraded, there is a cascade of effects from
incoherent information transfer, chaotic resonance
frequencies that undermine our own body's
synchronistic vibrational patterns, and an increase in the
rate of development of *de-structured energies and
environments.* This is electrically destroying and
contaminating our morphogenetic fields, which carry the
information our DNA doesn't have for our survival –
the collective consciousness field that has an impact on

the individual, their development, and their DNA expressions.

Insights into the structure of water and the functions and effects of structured water within our bodies give additional methods to understanding the dynamics of structured energetics. One crucial aspect of structured water, although rarely discussed, is the necessary structuring of the water within our bodies in order for our cells and tissues to even *use* the water. As we will see in the next chapter, all of the water within our bodies *must* have a specific structure in order to operate at an optimum state. Science can now show that the DNA in our bodies is literally encased in and surrounded by liquid water crystals that are structured in complex, sacred geometrical form – called sacred because they are shapes revered across cultures throughout antiquity. Researchers have also observed that when our water molecules are structured in a less perfect form, the DNA strands begin to degrade. Thus, our body attempts to restructure, as best it can, given its own energetic health and vibrational frequency, the de-structured water that it receives. Unfortunately, *it takes more energy for the body to restructure water than it receives from the water itself.* This means that as the body expends massive amounts of energy to restructure its water, the water it gets from this process is not enough to restore the energetic capacities it took to structure it. Thus, our body energetic storehouses and ability to carry out its processes are not restored back to optimal capacity *and the ability of the body to carry out its energetic processes begins a state of decline, and experiences an accelerating state of entropy and decay.* The crystalline structure that we are *supposed* to have in our environments lends towards states of non-entropy, observed in crystals, diamonds, and water, also called 'syntropic', meaning a cycle that breeds more life and higher states of organization. The structure of both the energetics of our natural environment *and* the water in our bodies are truly capable of and meant to support our systems towards *greater* Life.

# PART III

# WATER BEINGS

We have now explored how water functions as a liquid crystal, and how it can express different structures within the patterns of its molecular organization. We have seen how these different patterns within its structure affect its properties and characteristics, and how water physics demonstrate that all water is definitely not equal. We have also explored the mechanisms and implications of water's properties as a liquid crystal, which allows it to be dynamic and responsive to different forms of energetic stimuli. Having been introduced to new concepts and terms such as electromagnetic frequencies, coherence, fractals, and entropy, we are now able to understand the physics and potential implications of water as a liquid crystal, and can even apply these understandings to the deeper physical reality of our Universe as operating on a dynamic sea of energy that expresses characteristics similar to that of structured water, in terms of its fractal nature, responsiveness, and dependence upon primal geometric structures of pattern and organization. Now, let us further our exploration into structured water and structured energy as we take a deeper look into our physiology and bio-energetic systems as primarily structured water-based beings.

CHAPTER 11

# A REAL LOOK AT YOUR BODY'S
# WATER SYSTEM

---

*We stand as the manifested equivalent of three buckets of
water and a handful of minerals.*
~SAUL WILLIAMS
POET

*Be Water, my Friend.*
~BRUCE LEE

If we are to understand our physiology, how energy
and consciousness actually affects the physical systems,
and how to *repair* or even *truly prevent* dysfunctions in
the body that give rise to symptoms of illness, aging, and
disease, we *must* begin to view our bodies *as they actually
are* – disregarding our previous notions from science
textbooks and Biology 101 – and we must begin to
understand *what this reality means.*

*Organisms are so dynamically coherent at the molecular
level that they appear to be crystalline. There is a*

*dynamic, liquid crystalline continuum of connective tissues and extra cellular matrix linking directly into the equally liquid crystalline cytoplasm in the interior of every single cell in the body... Every part is in communication with every other part through a dynamic, tunable, responsive liquid crystalline medium that pervades the whole body, from organs and tissues to the interior of every cell.*

~DR. MAE WON HO
GENETICIST, PROFESSOR OF BIOPHYSICS
DIRECTOR: INSTITUTE OF SCIENCE IN
SOCIETY
OPEN UNIVERSITY, UK
CATANIA UNIVERSITY, SICILY

We are made almost completely of Structured Water, and composed primarily of crystalline structures – both solid crystals (i.e. bone, dentin) and liquid crystals (i.e. water, cellular membranes, collagen, fatty tissues, cell salts, cholesterols, enzymes, and proteins). **The structured water in our bodies acts as a fractal antenna, making possible our incredibly complex communicatory systems.**

Even by weight mass, we are approximately 90% water at birth, declining to 50-70% by death. Also by weight mass, 83% of the body's blood, 90% of the brain, and 90% of the body's nerves are water. As previously stated, more than 99% of the *molecules* in our body are *water*. And not just "any" water – our bio-water, the water within our bodies, is highly structured. Everywhere water is found in the body – which is, virtually, everywhere – it is found to exist in a state of complex, geometrically ordered molecular lattices and arrangements, giving it the fractal antenna properties on which our physical, emotional, mental, energetic, and consciousness systems depend on for health and proper functioning.

> *The roughly 10 layers of water molecules that can fit into these spaces [within the cell] have entirely different properties from water in "bulk"... Water as we know it, that hydrogen-bonded bulk liquid melting at 0°C and boiling at 100°C, may not exist within cells.*
> ~DR. MARTINA HAVENITH
> GERMAN ACADEMY OF SCIENCES
> AUSTRIAN SCIENCE COUNCIL
> CHAIR OF PHYSICAL CHEMISTRY
> RUHUR UNIVERSITY, GERMANY

The average human cell is at least 70% water by weight. Because water molecules are so small, that 70% weight represents more than 99% of the molecules in the cell – a mirror image of the water in the human body, representing roughly 70 % mass and more than 99% of the molecules, and adhering to the old adage of "as above, so below (and everywhere in between)." Within the cell, the structure of the water is responsible for the structural integrity of the cell itself, forming and maintaining the cellular membrane, as well as transmitting and decoding electromagnetic fields and frequencies. It is vital to the energy production and metabolism of the cell, and in delivering nutrients and removing toxins. In the brain and nervous system, nerve transmission is highly dependent upon water, as the electrical signals throughout the nervous system travel along a complex and elaborate system of small waterways, containing a fluid made up primarily of water and some conductive minerals. Messenger proteins, called transporter proteins, travel at lightning speeds within this water medium, delivering messages to every cell and organ in our body. The brain is completely bathed in a 99% water solution called cerebrospinal fluid, which also flows in and around the spine as part of the central nervous system.

Of course, this is not simple bulk water that is bathing our brain or maintaining our cellular integrity – it is highly structured water. In order for information to be transferred in our body, it has to travel at incredible speeds and the information has to reach its destination intact, otherwise our brain, endocrine, and cardiovascular system run the risk of receiving improper or mixed up messages and becoming unable of maintaining our system. In order to achieve this feat, our body uses its liquid crystal network system, which allows for incredibly reliable and fast information transfer.

Our liquid crystal network system is the amazing magic that allows us to exist and our bodies to persist. Energy, and thus information, is efficiently conducted along the complex crystalline structures and geometrically precise arrangements of our liquid crystal system. All parts of the network are interlaced and primarily made of structured water, which is vibrating in harmonic resonant frequencies. Because they are all vibrating in resonance to each other, information is efficiently processed. Resonance allows for an energetic dialogue, wherein the various components exchanging energy and information are able to essentially 'speak the same language' and not experience 'mistranslations' in the information transfer. Our complex physiological systems require this type of effective and efficient energy and information transfer in the body, for even slight mistranslations could mean our internal body temperature is not properly regulated, or our heart and cardiovascular system not responsive to the body's needs during exercise or stress. The human body could not persist, much less be a dominant species, without this complex network that allows for such quality and speed of information transfer.

Water has many functions in the body, including playing an important part in the liquid crystal cellular membrane (the envelope around every cell, through which all things entering and exiting the cell goes). Water also plays a vital role in energetic transduction (converting one form of energy or signal to another), information transfer, and frequency communication. Earlier we described the power of our cells in utilizing electromagnetic frequencies to communicate, transferring information and responding to fluctuations in the body's internal and external environment. It is well known that cells and organs decode electromagnetic frequencies and alter their frequency or initialize cellular processes in response, however it is much less well known *how* the cell is able to operate such complex informational processing and computing – the cell's 'nucleic brain' does not account for such activity. Rather, it is the *water* that performs this computing power, water inside and outside the cell, as well as in the liquid crystal cellular membrane, which is responsible for the decoding and transmitting electromagnetic frequencies and operates as a fractal antenna system to receive and transmit information. Every molecule that approaches the cell is surrounded by water, the cell itself is comprised mostly of water, and every cellular interaction happens in, and through, water. Acting in the body as the incredible solvent it is in nature, it utilizes the electrical properties of cellular salts and ions with its highly structured state to conduct information at lightning fast speeds. It restructures in response to incoming information and energy in the form of electromagnetic frequencies, thus altering the activity of the cell while creating and managing the natural fluctuations of its own electromagnetic frequency. The water in the cell manages a complex system of natural fluctuations, which mediate cellular response and signals while maintaining harmony and synchronization with the body's many nesting frequencies. It is also the body's natural defense system against interfering electromagnetic frequencies that we might normally encounter in nature. The highly structured water is designed to maintain the cell's structural integrity and a high level of functioning within the entire organism, independent of external electromagnetic activity. Frequencies are received, decoded, and processed by the body's water system, and when these frequencies are negative and damaging, it protects us from immediate disruption by adjusting its structural pattern so as to still achieve the desired function of the cellular processes. Because of its inherent memory and information storage however, the effect of a negative frequency is still expressed in the structure of the water, which has now experienced a level of disorder or de-structuring within its pattern, much like a weakened immune system. Also like an immune system, after persistent or excessive exposure (excessive in terms of either the level of electromagnetic frequency or frequencies, or the duration or intensity of exposure), the water becomes de-structured to such a degree that pathology or dis-ease begins to result.

These complex systems were developed to defend against interfering electromagnetic activity we might encounter in nature – our exposure to artificial electromagnetic frequencies is a recent development in human history and we are clearly not adapted for it, as the evidence of their serious dangers suggest. In our physiological systems, the level of the water's structure is truly all that matters. If the water in our bodies becomes de-structured to the degree that symptoms of dis-ease results and is not at least partially corrected, then a cycle of entropy will begin to be established. This means that the water begins a feedback loop of increasingly degrading structure and greater symptoms of disease, which in turn cause disruptions in the larger system, disruptions which in turn cause greater dis-ease and symptoms of disorder – the literal physics behind the "downward spiral" of degrading health.

Knowing that our physiology is actually *water-based* and not merely mechanistic allows us greater insight into other aspects of the body. When we approach our biology and physiology in this way, we begin to see the real role our systems and organs play in our health and development. This is particularly true of the heart, which is perhaps Western medicine's most confusing organ. The heart has long been perceived in a mechanistic function, its purpose denigrated to that of a mere blood pump. And yet, the main purpose of the heart is *not* to pump the blood. The heart, in fact, *does not pump blood, nor does it have the capacity to do so.* Embryonic studies show that the blood begins to circulate before the heart has even developed sufficiently, an observation that automatically negates the role of the heart as a necessary 'pump'. Rather than *pumping* the blood (which would take a much larger and stronger muscle than the heart in order to overcome gravity and atmospheric pressure), the heart actually *vortexes the blood around a vacuum of space.*[1] This is a radical shift in thinking, as we realize that rather than pumping

1. Buhner, Stephen Harrod. 2004.

blood throughout our vascular system like water through a hose, the heart actually *twists* our bloodstream and vortexes it through the vascular system much more like water vortexes down a flushing toilet or spirals down a whirlpool. In our *real* physiology, our blood is actually divided into three separate streams that are twisted, braided, and intertwined, projected out of our heart in this woven manner, and sent coursing throughout our body around a vacuum of empty space within each of our veins and arteries. This phenomenon – the twisting, braiding, and vortexing of our blood, can only be observed in *living tissue,* as the vacuum of space in the middle of our veins and arteries rapidly collapses when the spark of life has left the body. This is what gave scientists the impression that our vascular system was more like a pumping water hose and less like a twisting vortexing toilet, for before the recent technological advancements that allow us to observe the way the blood is actually flowing in living organisms and tissue, our understandings of the body's internal physiology and anatomy was heavily dependent upon autopsy-based investigations. Today's advancements have allowed us a glimpse at the amazing wonder of the living body, and it is even more extraordinary and incredible than we once believed.[2]

This revelation of the body's internal mechanics gives great insight into the intelligence of the body in regards to electromagnetic fields and structuring capacities. We know that the blood is composed mostly of water and other liquid crystal components, as well as magnetic materials in the form of iron (i.e. hemoglobin, magnetite). We also know that *vortexing* water generates an electromagnetic field, and that this also affects the

2. Buhner, Stephen Harrod. 2004.

structure of water. Thus, we can begin to see that as our blood is braided and vortexes through the twisting action of the heart around a vacuum of space throughout our vascular system, this surging vortex of liquid crystals and magnetics in highly conductive and electrically charged fluids generates an electromagnetic field that contributes to the structure of its liquid crystal components (which comprises over 83% of the blood, by weight). This is an important biological understanding, and provides us with some knowledge regarding some of the methods the body uses to affect its liquid crystal fluid system. The body, in its incredibly complex and sophisticated design, doesn't just depend on the elaborate arrangement and network of geometrically precise flexible structured water for its processes – it also has beautifully advanced and intricate systems in place to help maintain them.

It has to be maintained if we are to live at all – particularly when the effect that the structure of our water has on the development, maintenance, and expression of DNA is incalculable. Today, we know that the DNA strand is **surrounded and encased** by layers of structured water, and that it has a pillar of structured water layers through its central column.[3] We also know that it is the relationship between the DNA and the structured water surrounding it that is responsible for the DNA's coiling, its conduction of lightening fast resonant frequency communications, the coherency of its electromagnetic field, and *even its genetic information.* Scientists already discovered that "the precise DNA structure depends on the specific water surrounding the molecule"[4], and that the structure of the water

3. Samal S, Geckeler KE. Unexpected Solute Aggregation in Water on Dilution. Journal of Chemical Communications, 2001 Nov 7; (21):2224-5.
4. Hassan Khesbak, Olesya Savchuk, Satoru Tsushima, Karim Fahmy. The Role

surrounding proteins, and DNA, *determines the ultimate expression of shape that protein or DNA exhibits,* which in turn determines its function. They are already putting this knowledge to experimental use, successfully altering the genetic expression of salmon DNA by manipulating, or changing, the water surrounding it.[5]

> *Water molecules surround the genetic material DNA in a very specific way...[and] actually influences the structure of the genetic substance itself...The precise DNA structure depends on the specific amount water surrounding the molecule...*
>
> ~DR. CHRISTINE BOHNET
> HELMHOLTZ ASSOCIATION OF GERMAN
> RESEARCH CENTRES

The waters surrounding and within the DNA strands are also responsible for its conduction, again transferring and conducting this information at lightning speeds via resonant frequency communication. It is also responsible for maintaining the DNA's structure and stability, as well as maintaining the coherency of its electromagnetic field. *The level to which the water conducts and supports the DNA, and its corresponding electromagnetic field, is directly related to the geometric complexity of its structure.* Additionally, it has been found that the structure of the water surrounding proteins and DNA *determines the ultimate expression of shape that protein or DNA exhibits.* In fact *all* of the components in cells are dissolved in water, and derive their structure and activity from their interactions with the water.[6] Earlier we discussed how it is really the

of Water H-Bond Imbalances in B-DNA Substate Transitions and Peptide Recognition Revealed by Time-Resolved FTIR Spectroscopy. *Journal of the American Chemical Society,* 2011; 133 (15): 5834

5. Hassan Khesbak, et al. 2011.

*structure* of the protein, rather than the ingredients itself, which determines how the protein functions. Now we know what is responsible for the structure of the protein – the water surrounding it. And just like proteins, the same holds true for DNA, which as we know is a much more malleable and non-static than previously believed, capable even of changing in response to its environment, which actually occurs as a result of its response to the change in the structure of the water surrounding it.

This has been demonstrated through the findings that *healthy* DNA is surrounded by water in a highly structured, geometrically complex form of molecular arrangement, whereas *unhealthy* DNA is encased in water that exhibits *less* geometric complexity.[7] [8] The higher the complexity of the structure, the stronger the electromagnetic field, which indicates higher energy potential and information transfer as well as greater efficiency and cellular function. In other words: the greater the structure, the greater the health.

Conversely, the lower the structure of the water, the greater the disorder of the physical system and what we would call "ill health". Here, we see that a more entropic structure – one with less geometric complexity, symmetry, and structural integrity – results in greater and more rapid decay. Less geometric complexity in the water surrounding the DNA means a weaker electromagnetic field, reduced cellular function, and alterations in the structural expression of the double helix – which are sometimes called mutations and can lead to

6. Kumar Pal, Samir, Zhao, Liang, and Zewail, Ahmed. Water at DNA surfaces: Ultrafast dynamics in minor groove recognition. Proceedings of the National Academy of Sciences of the United States of America, 2003 May 21; (vol 100, 14) 8113-8118.
7. Thayer, Jeff. *The DNA and Structured Water Interfaces.* 2011.
8. Jhon, M.S. *The Water Puzzle and the Hexagonal Key.* Uplifting Press, Inc. 2004.

the development of cancerous cells. It also means there is an *accelerated degradation of the DNA strand*, which can also be recognized as *accelerated aging*. In water's great responsiveness as a liquid crystal to change its geometric structure to incorporate new information, the crystalline structure degrades with exposure to environmental pollution, toxins, mental and emotional distress, and through not being hydrated with properly structured water. Thus, over time the integrity of the DNA strand is compromised. The telomeres on the ends of the DNA begin to fray and break apart during replications, which we experience as aging. The *telomeres*, which are similar to long fibers on the end of the DNA, become shorter and more frayed with every replication. After 120 years or so of DNA replication, the fibers are typically frayed to the end and a person experiences "death by old age", leading scientists to often consider telomeres as the 'age-marker' for DNA. The rate at which the fibers are fraying can indicate an individual's life-expectancy based on the health of their telomeres. Of course, many factors contribute to accelerated aging, and the quality of life and environmental toxin exposures are major contributors. Exposure to toxins – whether physical toxins or emotional and consciousness toxins – can cause a more rapid decay of the telomere fibers. It does so by affecting the structural integrity of the body's water system, which in turn is responsible for the expression, health, and integrity of the DNA strand and its fibrous ends. Entropic water structures – those that have reduced levels of organization and intelligent arrangement – lack the sufficient structural integrity to maintain the healthy expression of the DNA. This is expressed in the decline of the DNA's structural health – which we experience as *aging*.

# CHAPTER 12

# AGING AND DEHYDRATION

*Aging is a phenomenon of our body becoming gradually drier.*
~DR. ISHIHARI YUMI, M.D.

Aging, the experience of entropy in the human body and the degrading function of physical systems, has a special relationship to dehydration. Not only is aging accompanied by dehydration, researchers have also found that the water remaining has experienced substantial changes in its structural formation.[1] This has allowed us to see that changes in the structure of the bio-water, namely a loss of geometric complexity and symmetry, have *a direct relationship* to dehydration and aging. The critical functions and capacities of bio-water in cellular and systemic communication, nutrient delivery and toxin elimination, the movement of molecules, and diffusion (the ability of water to cross membranes) all decline with age. We may even experience an increase in our extra-cellular fluids, or the fluid between cells, but it is not significantly structured to permeate cell walls and can

1. Brodskaga, EN. Molecular dynamics investigation of the structure of water microclusters. Leningrad U. Kolloidin Zh. 1986; 48(1): 3-16.

instead collect in undesirable places, causing edema. In order to permeate the cell and be sufficiently hydrating for the body – allowing it to perform the necessary functions of the cell – it must be sufficiently structured. Thus, structured water science shows us that aging is truly the result of loss of structure in the bio-water, which is the root cause of the dehydration associated with aging and its related effects of physical decay.

A number of books have been written on the subject of dehydration as the cause of aging, and the adage of "dying of old age," being essentially death by dehydration. These books tout the cure for aging as drinking more water, and if all water were equal then this would be true. As we have well seen by now, all water is definitely not equal in quality or properties, and the water inside of the body responsible for our level of youth or rate of aging is quite a different substance from the eight glasses of water we are told to drink every day. While eight daily glasses are by no means a cure for aging, overcoming cellular dehydration certainly is.

> *The cell is immortal. It is merely the fluid in which it floats that degenerates. Renew this fluid at regular intervals, give the cells what they require for nutrition, and as far as we know, the pulsation of life can go on forever.*
> ~DR. ALEXIS CARREL
> NOBEL PRIZE, PHYSIOLOGY OR MEDICINE

Chronic low-grade dehydration (versus acute and clinical dehydration) affects nearly *everyone,* and increases in areas with greater pollution. Studies show that over 75% of people are chronically dehydrated, which is a conservative estimate. Compounding the issue is that subclinical dehydration doesn't necessarily trigger thirst

– in at least 37% of North Americans the thirst
mechanism has become so weak that dehydration is
mistaken for hunger, and as we age it weakens as well.[2]
Perhaps the reason for the weakening of our thirst
mechanism is because the issue is not the *quantity* of
water, it is the *quality*. In today's massively polluted
societies, where very few of our water sources are highly
structured and our bodies' bio-waters are becoming de-
structured as well, it is possible that the thirst mechanism
is not being triggered because the body has become
trained to recognize that what it gets in response to
triggering thirst – whether it is soda, juice, energy drinks,
bottled water, or water from the tap – does not fulfill
the body's need for highly structured fluids, and thus
weakens the mechanism through negative conditioning
rather than strengthening it through positive
reinforcement. Another possible theory is that the
massive process of de-structurization through
environmental and electromagnetic contaminations is
affecting the bio-waters of so many individuals in such
a way that eventually reaches a point of entropy where
the lack of thirst mechanism is simply another expression
of its state of decay and downward spiral, and the
expression of the natural principle of states of decay
persisting decay, the 'like attracts like' of the Law of
Attraction.

The weakening of our thirst mechanism, however, is
not the cause of chronic dehydration, the de-structuring
of our bio-waters is. As we lose structural integrity of our
bio-waters, we experience an increase in surface tension
that changes the properties of the water's permeability,

2. Kleiner, SM. Water: an essential but overlooked nutrient. *Journal of the
American Dietetics Association*. 1999;99(2):200-6. Available from: US National
Library of Medicine. Accessed February 14, 2013.

affecting its ability to enter or exit a cell, as well as changes in pH and a loss of coherence in the electromagnetic system. In order for the water in our bodies to be properly hydrating and capable of feeding our biological system the type of water it requires for proper function, it *must* be highly structured. Babies when they are born are approximately 90-95% water *by weight*, and it is highly structured, and the decline to 50-70% by the end of the average lifespan is really merely reflective of the level of de-structurization we experience throughout the course of our lives.

Research has shown that chronic dehydration is the root cause of many diseases associated with aging, including arthritis, GI disorders, and senile dementia. It also been observed that the structure of the bio-waters is directly related to the internal temperature of the body and its organs, as evident by its surface tension (which directly relates to its permeability), viscosity, and electrical conductivity. This explains why "snowbirds" move south during the winter to help with arthritis and other symptoms associated with aging. Their bio-waters are able to structure to higher form with a warmer internal environment, and as a result this dramatically affects their health. Other symptoms of aging, including the loss of skin tone and flexibility, the appearance of wrinkles, the reduction in firing patterns and brainwave coherence, and the decay of proteins related to Alzheimer's and other age-related disease, are all the result of the loss of structural integrity in the water system, which in fact is responsible for all of these things. The decline in eyesight that is so common with aging is also associated with dehydration; the lens of the eye is composed of 99% highly structured water, which maintains its flexibility (allowing for accurate and responsive changes in focus) and its strength of perception. It is also one of the first places the body draws from when requiring highly structured water for more critical cellular processes, and thus a loss of eyesight over time can often result in full blindness by the time the individual reaches elderly age. As we will discuss later, the structural integrity of the body's water system is also intimately related to *memory*, one of the classic casualties of aging and Alzheimer's.

There is quite disagreement amongst some scientists on whether aging is the result of dehydration or caused by the fraying and breaking apart of the DNA telomere strands, which they cite as a separate issue from dehydration. However, when one is knowledgeable of the critical role highly structured water plays in determining the shape, integrity, and electromagnetic field of the DNA, it is possible to recognize the connection between a loss of structure in the cellular fluids and a corresponding loss of integrity in the telomeres of the DNA. This connection is the important one to look at when trying to reduce the symptoms and expressions of aging, decrease accelerated aging processes, or increase longevity. When we realize that aging – and disease – are in fact by-products or *symptoms* of the loss of structure in our cellular fluids, and *not* the causative effect, we arrive at a more effective approach to treatment that is based on the actual mechanics of our biology. Aging does not cause de-structured bio-waters. De-structured bio-waters, rather, causes aging.

CHAPTER 13

# THE PROCESS OF
# DE-STRUCTURING

Since aging and disease are the *result* of de-structured bio-waters rather than the cause, as the research indicates, what *is* causing this loss of structure?

There are many sources of energetic stimuli and contamination that degrade the structural integrity and organization of our bio-water. The consciousness of the individual is perhaps the largest factor. The self-consciousness is responsible for both maintaining the body's Water structure as a living, loving, and spiritual conscious entity, and in degrading its structure as negative thought processes, confusion, stress, traumatic events, and overall accumulated emotional baggage become stored within the molecular structure of the individual's cellular fluids. We have seen demonstrations of this phenomena through the work of Emoto and Korotkov, who have both photographed the incredible loss of complexity and geometric form in ice crystals from water that has received negative thoughts, emotional toxins, and even negative inputs and polarizing images from our media and cultures. Not often considered, however, is the consciousness of the collective, which also has an effect on the structure of water – likely through the informational network of the energetic structures and morphogenetic fields of the planet. When we consider the incredible information and memory storage potential of water, we realize that negative thoughts, emotional toxins, and damaging inputs do not just affect us during the instant that we experience them, or those moments when we consciously recall them – they affect us all the time through the encoding of negative information into the structural patterns of our water, an essentially de-structuring or more entropic pattern, and through our constant sub-conscious awareness and memory, which is also intimately connected to our water system, as we will soon explore.

Of course physical toxins and pollutants de-structure water as well. This has also been visually demonstrated through the photography work of ice crystals exposed to pollutants, both physical chemicals and energetic toxins in the form of artificial EMF's. Harmful artificial electromagnetic frequencies degrade water's structural integrity; whether they are generated from computers, cell phones, televisions, radios, microwaves, Wi-Fi signals, or even the hum of your local power grid. They are coursing throughout the walls of our homes, occupying our environments in the form of radio frequencies, generated from our refrigerators, microwaves, televisions, electric blankets, baby monitors, GPS devices, iPads, and laptops (which should *never* be put on the lap). Even today's 'smartphones' come with a warning in their user's manual – *to keep the device at least one inch away from the body.* Which begs the question – if it is potentially dangerous to your health to even touch the device, how is a person supposed to use it? According to the safety instructions, smartphones should evidently be used entirely hands free. Holding smartphones next to your ear has been connected to brain tumors, cancers, and other diseases, through well-researched studies. Not because they are leaking a chemical poison – but because they are generating an electromagnetic one.

Everyday as our technological societies advance so does our increase in exposure to multiple forms of electromagnetic pollution, also known as 'electro-smog'. This topic is understandably controversial, with so much of society and a large branch of the economy having grown dependent upon the use and production of such technologies. Evidence continues to accumulate, however, which indicates that harmful – i.e. artificial and non-natural – electromagnetic frequencies have significant impacts on accelerated brain degeneration, tumors, and a host of mental and physical disorders. It is this kind of mounting data that has led to such actions as setting exposure limits or reductions, and requiring the removal of Wi-Fi from public schools in certain places throughout countries like Germany, Italy, France, India, Russia, Switzerland, Austria, Poland, Greece, Hungary, Israel, China, the United Kingdom, and Canada. In 2011 it caused the Council of Europe to recommend a full ban of Wi-Fi in schools throughout its 47 member countries, and prompted the World Health Organization to reclassify radiation from wireless devices and cellphones as a Class 2B possible carcinogen – the same class as lead, DDT, and car exhaust. The amassing evidence is also causing rising concerns among insurance companies over the potential increase in EMF related health claims over the coming years, as things such as cell phone use rises from an average of less than 3 hours per month to nearly 3 hours per day. The multitude of mental and physical disorders that those suffering from electromagnetic frequency pollution experience is a result of these dissonant, un-resonant frequencies. These degrade the structure of the body's water to such a degree that there begins a downward spiral of de-structuring bio-water and bio-energetic health disruption, eventually leading to the manifestation of physical symptoms and disease.

*There is currently enough evidence and technology available to warrant industry and governments alike in taking immediate steps to reduce exposure of consumers to mobile-phone related electromagnetic radiation and to make consumers clearly aware of potential dangers...*
~DR. VINI GAUTAM KHURANA (2008)
MAYO CLINIC TRAINED NEUROSURGEON

And yet, despite the voices of those like Dr. Khurana, the majority of consumers remain clueless and no steps are taken in our society to reduce exposure to mobile-phone related electromagnetic radiation. Government is heavily influenced by industry, and industry cares little for consumer health. When research demonstrated the negative effect the cellular phone's electromagnetic frequencies had on the fertility rates and health of peacocks and chickens, the response from a major phone company was, "We don't sell many phones to peacocks and chickens."[1] Until there is some kind of legal precedent, cell phone manufacturers and other high harmful EMF generating devices will continue to include their disclaimers in the fine print of their products, including the instructions and warnings to keep all smartphones at least one inch away from the body at all times. Industry is aware of the dangers, and yet continues to perpetuate consumer ignorance through

1. Blankenship, Joe. Personal Interview. 3 Feb. 2012.

advertisements and false marketing – there are few, if any, cell phone commercials that don't include someone holding and touching the phone, much less putting it to their head to talk. And yet this use of smartphones is against the safety instructions, which more or less suggest never actually physically touching your phone, since the high frequency electromagnetic energies emitted from such devices are linked to all kinds of diseases and cancers. It drives dehydration and structural destruction of the waters in the body, much in the same way it drives structural degradation in the photographic work by Korotkov, Emoto, and others. This de-structuring of our bio-waters in turn eventually manifests symptoms of disorder and disease in the body.

The effect of negative consciousness and harmful and artificial electromagnetic frequencies and radiations are not the only sources of water de-structurization, which occurs not only in our bio-waters but also in our drinking water through processing and delivery techniques, ozonation, distillation, and artificial ionization – all various 'water-purifying' practices. Many products are even marketing structured drinking water and structuring water devices that utilize electrolysis, another de-structuring process. During electrolysis the water is essentially electrocuted, breaking apart the hydrogen bonding that is so critical to its ability to function as a liquid crystal. While these waters may boast an increase in pH and decrease in surface tension, they do nothing to improve the structural form of the water bonds itself and rather degrade its crystallography instead, ripping it apart. Dr. Marcel Vogel, renowned crystallographer and the forefather of structured water science had this to say about electrolysis and the electrical process of ionization:

> *Ionization of the water can occur through structuring the water...or by electrical ionization... When the water is electrically ionized...the existing bonds in the water are torn apart... This process of ionization...creates water with an electrical charge, but with no structural charge. It does not have the structural information.*

Our municipal water systems are also contributing to the problem of degrading structure, using water delivery methods that de-structure our water and deliver a type of water to our entire population that is unsupportive to our life, our health, and our hydration. In nature, water *never* flows along a path of hard right angles, as it does in our piping systems. Rather, water flows along curving and winding paths that do not break apart its structure like traveling on a completely unnatural hard right angle will. As a result of our hard angle delivery systems, the water that reaches us in our faucet is de-structured due to delivery methods alone – much less its treatment process.

The treatment processes in our municipal water system involve primarily the use of chlorine as an anti-bacterial, fluoride as an additive, and a rock form of calcium (calcium carbonate) for pH stability. Calcium carbonate is added to make the water more basic and return it to an acceptable pH level due to the large amounts of chlorine we use which makes the water too acidic for consumption. There are other chemicals, additives, and constituents in the water coming from your tap, such as large amounts of "dissolved solids," (i.e. chemical and particulate 'sludge'), as well as chemicals and pharmaceuticals, particularly that of hormones and estrogen (primarily from the use of birth controls). This is why so many people use reverse osmosis filters or some other form of water treatment in their home – to remove the fluoride, chlorine, excessive calcium carbonate, pharmaceuticals, hormones, and other chemicals.

Proponents of chlorine, fluoride, and other water additives argue that the addition of harmful agents is required in order to make our drinking water 'safe' (with the exception of fluoride, which is added not for any anti-bacterial reason but under the guise of forced medication for a supposed dental health benefit). But this kind of extensive water treatment system, which involves the use of harmful and toxic agents, is completely unnecessary. Water has been treated with various frequencies and has been successfully made to exhibit anti-bacterial properties with *no* chemical additives. Harmful agents, including bacterium, parasites, pharmaceuticals, chlorine, and fluoride, can be made inert or completely removed by employing various water structuring methods, eliminating the need for chlorine or other such chemical treatments. The addition of fluoride to municipal water systems comes from the hazardous by-product of aluminum and fertilizer manufacturing, is added to the water in diluted form, and is a highly controversial issue. Against overwhelming evidence to the contrary, proponents of fluoride in drinking water contest that it is helpful for white teeth. On the other hand, opponents of fluoride cite numerous studies demonstrating the toxic and dangerous effects of its use in our drinking systems, its failure to aid dental health when ingested, and challenge the ethics of forced medicating through public water. Regardless who is right here (although at this point it is fairly obvious that adding fluoride to drinking water offers no benefit and great harm), both of these issues are resolved with structuring methods. If fluoride is indeed added to help our teeth (which are composed of dentin, a hard crystal), structured water treatments could potentially replace the "need" for fluoride in our water. If it is in fact an extremely dangerous chemical, as the evidence quite strongly suggests, then employing municipal and home re-structuring systems could either completely eliminate the fluoride or render its molecules inert – depending on the quality of the structuring methods being employed.

CHAPTER 14

# OTHER IMPLICATIONS AND APPLICATIONS

## FROM FARMING TO DESALINATION

While some of the implications and applications of structured water science have already been demonstrated, our focus so far has remained primarily on structured water as it relates to our internal water system, health, and the treatment of disease. But the potential applications of structured water science and the implications suggested by what research has already demonstrated are remarkable, and can be incorporated into a variety of disciplines and objectives, from medicine to agriculture. We have already discussed the effect structured water science can have on the field of medicine and disease treatment, and have explored the connections between cancer, diabetes, HIV, and other forms of disease – including multiple sclerosis, fibromyalgia, chronic pain, and chronic fatigue – with the de-structure of our bio-waters. As every system in our body is affected by the structure of our bio-waters, every system can potentially be treated using methods that correctly apply this knowledge. We have also already discussed the current research involving structured water for pharmaceutical preservation; structured water can also affect the preservation rates of substances and water-based foods and carries large implications in the quality, production, and preservation of food, fish, and meat.

The benefits of structured water science application in agriculture are fairly obvious, and are a subject that has been demonstrated and explored in research and experiments for decades. Structured water exhibits remarkable properties, and its effects on seed germination rates and plant growth, anti-bacterial properties, enzyme function, preservation rates, and DNA transference are just some examples of the wide range of potential applications involving structured water. Water is so central to life, society, and development; the ways in which it can be used for the benefit of our societies and our planet are limitless and the value its science can hold for humanity is incalculable.

In agricultural applications, studies published in reputable scientific journals have demonstrated **a five-fold increase in root elongation, accelerated seed germination, increases in the health and rate of growth of plants, accelerated fruiting and ripening processes, and higher yields.** Other research indicates higher concentrations of vitamins and anti-oxidants, a decreased need for fertilizers and pesticides, stronger plant resilience to disease and insects, longer preservation times, and better drought tolerance – i.e. requiring less water for growth and fruiting. Fruits and vegetables that are watered with structured water retain their integrity much longer than "bulk-watered" fruits, lasting much longer before spoiling, indicating that the vitamins, minerals, anti-oxidants and other beneficial phytochemicals are not decomposing at the same rate of bulk-watered produce, which break down rapidly after being picked. Keeping produce from rotting too quickly off of the vine is one of the main reasons it is sprayed with chemical waxes and preservatives before being shipped to supermarkets all over the country. And while too little research has been done on the use of structured water in the raising of livestock, it is logical to assume that there would be significant increase in the health of the animals and the quality of their respective products or meat, as has been reported already by several farmers. It is equally logical to presume that supplying animals with structured water would increase their lifespan and reduce diseases, as well as cause a substantially reduced need for agricultural pharmaceuticals and steroids, or 'growth-promoters', and that this same principle can be applied to the water used in fisheries. At this point, the research revealing the dangers of genetically-modified foods, chemical pesticides, herbicides, chemical preservatives, insecticides, and fertilizers are well known, and come with a growing multitude of correlating diseases including cancers, Alzheimer's, Parkinson's, neurological imbalances and mental illnesses, skin diseases, digestive and intestinal disorders, and toxicity reactions, which has led to a massive movement towards organic foods and farming. Structured water can and should be a vital part of any organic farming operation, much less every farming operation.

The above-mentioned recognized benefits of structured water in farming are just the beginning of a rapidly expanding list, as more people begin to investigate the effects and potentials of using structured water within this field. It is impossible at this point to measure the benefits that small or large-scale structured water agricultural applications might have on the environment and the health of our communities. We use massive amounts of water in our agriculture practices, and in a time where areas are becoming more arid and water sources are drying up, the ability to enhance the water so that less of it is required by crops is going to be an *incredible* asset. Considering the water shortages and restrictions already experienced by so much of the United States and the world, the use of structured water in large-scale agriculture should already be a common practice. Why such methods are not regularly employed today can only be the result of ignorance, supported by the dominating forces of massive corporate farms, chemical companies, and the pharmaceutical industries who continue to profit from the consequences of chemically based farming practices using bulk or de-structured water instead of contributing fruitful, sustainable, healthy, and sound ecological practices. Rather, much of our agriculture employs damaging and destructive practices, at great cost to the quality and production of our food as well as our own health and the health of our planet.

One of the other obvious potential applications of structured water science involves reversing the effects of pollution, and providing successful and effective ecological cleanup solutions. Structured water and structuring processes can be used to render contaminants inert, if not completely eliminate them.[1] In a time when our ecological system suffers more damage and a higher level of pollution than it has ever before experienced, with no sign of slowing down, these types of technological developments are absolutely critical.

But perhaps the most compelling application of

1. Mikesell, N. *The Mikesell Research Papers: The Work of Norman deLauder Mikesell on Structured Water and Cellular Biology.* 1995.

structured water science, besides of course physical health, aging, and in the treatment of virtually every disease and illness, is in the world of water purification, desalination (removing salt from water), and water transportation. These are the most challenging issues facing those trying to solve the world's water crisis. As of 2005, over one billion people in developing nations did not have access to safe drinking water, a fact largely responsible for the current state of most of the world's impoverished, malnourished, and disease-ridden communities.[2] Billions of dollars in research have been spent to devise ways to bring fresh water to such communities, while public water sources in these areas are being bought and run by privatized companies who are then charging access. Additional agriculture and industry water demands are predicted to double by 2050 in order to cope with the needs of projected population increases. In order to begin to solve the world's current water crisis as well as prevent even greater ones in the future, new approaches involving structured water principles will be necessary.

*We need a new global culture that finds the existence of millions of thirsty people thoroughly and immediately unacceptable... We have the ability to provide clean water for every man, woman and child on the Earth. What has been lacking is the collective will to accomplish this. What are we waiting for?*

~JEAN-MICHEL COUSTEAU
PRESIDENT OCEAN FUTURES SOCIETY

---

2. World Health Organization/UNICEF. *Joint Monitoring Programme for Water Supply and Sanitation, Water for Life: Making it Happen.* Geneva, Switzerland: WHO Press, 2005.

SON OF OCEAN EXPLORER JACQUES
COUSTEAU

As previously stated, this issue is three-fold. Water purification is absolutely necessary – many areas have access to fresh water, but not clean and safe drinking water. Water transportation is key – fresh water is not equally distributed on the planet, instead some regions have an abundance of water, or even too much, while others experience a dire need. *Desalination*, or the process of removing salt from water (i.e. turning sea water to fresh water), would be the world's ultimate achievement in bringing an end to the world's water crisis: over 98% of the water on Earth is in the oceans, with only .003% available for drinking, hygiene, agriculture, and industry – a figure that includes the fresh water sources in the polar ice caps and other inaccessible regions, making the actual percentage of freshwater available (and accessible) for drinking, hygiene, agriculture, and industry closer to .0007% of the Earth's water.[3] This is a staggering number, and with the overwhelming majority of the world's water locked in the seas, one can quickly grasp the value of desalination methods to support the world's current and growing water needs.

The implications of structured water science emphatically imply that these three challenges in providing quality water access for all can be solved by developing and applying advanced structuring techniques. As mentioned in our discussion on municipal water sources, water-structuring processes have remarkable effects on the purity of the water. In some

3. Food and Agriculture Organization of the United Nations. Crops and Drops: Making the Best Use of Water for Agriculture. World Food Day. Rome, Italy: FAO, 2002.

cases, water that has been structured by various methods exhibits a complete removal of harmful chemical compounds and contaminates, while other times it shows a drastic reduction in concentration levels. Additionally, chemical compounds and harmful substances such as chlorine and fluoride are rendered inert in certain structuring methods, drastically reducing or even eliminating their harmful effects in the body.[4] The Russian military has been purifying their water by filtering it through *shungite,* a carbon-based mineral, which purifies the water by re-structuring it as it is poured over the rocks. Scientists at the St. Petersburg University have confirmed shungite's ability to remove toxic components like chlorine, pesticides, and heavy metals, while improving the water's quality, essential mineral levels, and anti-oxidant potentials.[5]

The research that has been conducted to study the potentials of structuring water for purification purposes is incredibly promising, and does more than just hint at the possibility of ending such global hardship, especially when it begins to involve the potentials of desalination processes. Outside of the implications of structured water for disease treatment and preventative health care, desalination perhaps the most compelling implication of structured water science. Using structuring techniques to purify already fresh water is amazing in itself, but if we were able to engage such processes to achieve the desalination, or a 'de-salting', of seawater in order to turn it into fresh and drinkable water, it would be one of mankind's greatest achievements in supporting both the

4. Mikesell, N. *The Mikesell Research Papers: The Work of Norman deLauder Mikesell on Structured Water and Cellular Biology.* 1995.
5. Selinus O., Finkelman R.B. and Centeno, J.A. Medical Geology: A Regional Synthesis. Springer, 2010.

needs of our environment and our global family community. Societies would no longer have to worry about fresh water sources and the perils associated with limited or insufficient access, which claim *millions* of lives every year. The typical methods employed today to achieve desalination are incredibly inefficient, but the potentials of using sea water in specific structuring methods that are targeted at releasing the salt from its chemical bonds are extremely promising. Desalination structuring methods would likely involve the use of water-resonance, vortex principles, and natural frequency stimulation (as opposed to electric frequency stimulation, which is de-structuring rather than re-structuring). By restructuring the salt water using the appropriate techniques, the salt can be separated from the water, creating a fresh, drinkable water source.

Technologies and developments are already in the works to apply water-structuring methods for purification and desalination purposes, and more are sure to follow. Reaching farther than the obvious applications in these two areas, we realize just how much we could achieve by developing advanced structuring methods when we consider aspects *water transportation,* which involves carrying large amounts of water over long distances, one of the great challenges in providing clean water to those in need. The implications structured water has on the ability to transport water is something that seems to have gone completely unnoticed. This is perhaps because the implication alone is an incredible paradigm shifter, and requires thinking outside the box of modern physics in order to operate in the natural world and microcosmic natural order. It is not unreasonable, rather it is perfectly logical, that structuring methods and science could become advanced enough to create very specific types of bonding, structuring, and nesting of water molecules. With this type of technology, it is reasonable to suggest that water could be structured to condense its molecules into geometries that are more nested, or more tightly folded into each other – allowing for a compression and condensing of water into smaller volume for transportation that could then be structured to expand its molecules once it has reached its destination point, growing in volume back to its original state.

The possibilities for what can be achieved through applying structured water principles for the betterment of humanity are endless, and things such as water purification systems, agriculture applications, ecological cleanup solutions, and disease treatment and prevention are just the beginning. These are just the tip of the iceberg of what can be accomplished by employing these principles. Later, as we examine the link between consciousness and the structural systems of our bio-waters, we shall see the implications that structured bio-water treatments may hold for the fields of psychology, human behavior, and psychiatry. The connection between an individual's water system and their corresponding consciousness and mental patterns is highly suggestive of a powerful new approach to treating the currently evasive root cause of these symptoms of imbalance. To be able to treat both physical illness and psychological illness through the water of the body is something we should view as the most practical, useful, and effective approach to solving these challenging problems. This approach applies to all forms of mental illness, including depression, anxiety, autism, Alzheimer's, and Asperger's. Structured bio-water treatments could also be developed to apply towards all types behavioral disorders, including all forms of emotional and behavioral disabilities, attention deficit disorders, and learning disabilities. Because the structure of the water surrounding the DNA is actually responsible for the structure of the genetic information – which is entirely *structure* based and not reliantly *code* based as generally believed (recall it is the structure that determines the information, not the chemical make-up, and that it is the water surrounding the DNA, as well as every other protein and molecule in the body, that determines its structure and how it functions). Developing treatments targeted at affecting the structure of the water surrounding the DNA to repair defects could potentially be the most successful approach to this type of disease treatment.

But in order to employ these types of solutions and treatments using principles of structured water, we must have a solid understanding of the rest of our *real* water system. This requires a certain level of examination regarding the relationship between water, consciousness, and memory, as well as how our subtle energy and bio-energetic systems relate to water. Only then can we grasp how water acts as an interface, translating subtle energy information into manifested physical form. Only then are we capable of answering that most difficult question of *how* to affect the structure of our bio-water for our greatest benefit, and fully grasp how Water can hold the seat of our consciousness.

# CHAPTER 15

# YOUR CONSCIOUSNESS AND MEMORY: YOUR WATER SYSTEM

---

*In many cases [of cultural history], water appears as a
reflection or an image of the Soul.*
~DR. CHRISTOPHER WITCOMBE
PROFESSOR OF ART HISTORY

*Looking for consciousness in the brain is like looking inside
a radio for the announcer.*
~NASSIM HARAMEIN

For all of its advancements, today's science and
technology *still* cannot tell us definitively where memory
is stored, much less where our consciousness is. Through
understanding the science of structured water, we can
come to understand not only where, but also *how* our
consciousness and memory are stored. We can also begin
to comprehend the sacred teachings and secrets
surrounding pervasive concepts across multiple religions,
to gain a complete and holistic understanding of what
water *really is, really does,* and *really can do.*

So where are consciousness and memory stored? How

does it all work, why does it affect our physical systems so greatly? These questions have been asked and studied by the greatest minds around the world for centuries, and with advanced modern equipment for decades, and still no one has been able to provide definitive information or workable model. Yet two of the most primary phenomena examined by scientists, philosophers, and theologians throughout antiquity correlate exactly with structured water model.

In the search for the location of memory, one of the most studied and fascinating phenomena are the numerous documented cases where patients and individuals have an accurate memory of an experience that occurred *without* proper brain function. Many patients under intense anesthesia, undergoing brain surgery, or even while pronounced dead, have reported clear and accurate memory of events that happened to and around them during these states. Even when all vitals are failed and there is *no* electrical activity associated with conscious or life processes in the body, prior to being revived or coming back to life, some patients have *still* accurately described things that were said or happened to and around them, even without any of the brain activity we would normally deem "necessary" for proper memory information storage.

For decades scientists have tried to answer the questions this phenomenon raises – *how* is this possible, and if brain activity is *not* necessary or even responsible for memory information storage as the phenomenon suggests, *what is?* And because the *memory* of our experiences (and our associated reactions to them) is such a critical part of our definition of our *consciousness,* as it represents our relationship to *who we are* (as a collection of self-relevant thoughts and memories), what does the

location and operation methods of our memory reveal
about the "location" and "operation methods" of our
consciousness?

For one well versed in the properties and capabilities of
structured water, the answer is obvious, for the capacity
for information, energy, and the necessary *responsiveness*
to encode information (i.e. memory storage), is *infinite*
within the realm of structured bio-water. While the
number of cells in our body is an ever-growing number
as science develops more accurate methods of
measurement, let us use some relatively accepted figures
to put the potentials of information storage in the body's
water system into perspective:

> Assuming there are roughly **50 trillion cells** in the
> average human body (not counting bacteria cells),
> with approximately *23 trillion molecules per cell,* **99%**
> **of which are composed of structured water** – we
> arrive at a number near one thousand trillion trillion
> molecules of structured water in the average human
> body, or 1,000,000,000,000,000,000,000,000,000.[1] By
> some measurements, which put the number of cells
> in the human body closer to 100 trillion, this number
> would be doubled – one thousand trillion trillion x 2.
> Recall that water molecules are found structured into
> clusters, and that each cluster holds *at least* 440,000
> *different panels* for information storage. Again doing
> the math, we realize that we can estimate a staggering
> potential                                              of
> *440,000,000,000,000,000,000,000,000,000,000* panels of
> information storage within the bio-water of the
> average person, a number potentially doubled based

---

1. University of California Santa Barbara and National Science Foundation.
   *Science Line.* Web. 2014.

on conflicting estimates of cells within the body. This does not even tell us how much information each *panel* is capable of containing. When we start looking at the numbers, they grow very fast, very quickly – and that's **before** we take the fractality of water into consideration, which already suggests an infinite nature of information capacity.

Thus, we understand that since water is *responsive* – intelligently encoding the energy to which it is exposed as information within its structural arrangement – and since this responsiveness is *immediate,* and the energy and information is encoded in its structure *independently of biological processes,* we can see that the water in the human body has the capacity to store the information of memory in a highly organized fashion that can later be retrieved and processed by the brain. Thus, memory *is* non-local, as science has described, being found not in one particular region of the brain or body but rather spread throughout the intense and complex network of our body's water and liquid crystal systems as information stored in within their geometric patterns. But it's not just our memory – **it's our entire consciousness**.

While trying to find the location of consciousness, scientists have tried to locate a *specific point of activity* that initiates the cascade of physical reactions our bodies experience in response to a thought. The idea is that what we term our consciousness expresses itself in *thought,* and that by finding what makes our *thoughts* we will also find the seat of consciousness, the bridge to the sub-conscious, and the potential storehouse of our 'soul' or 'spirit'. Certainly for decades, if not centuries, it was assumed that this initial spark of 'thought' most likely occurred in the brain or even the heart. No matter where it was, it was most certainly believed to start from some initial, localized point of thought-generation. Instead, to the surprise and vexation of many scientists, what studies have revealed is that the response in the body's *many* systems – expressed as electrical changes in the brain, fluctuations in the electromagnetic field of the heart, stimulated processes in the immune and endocrine system, etc. – all experience these changes *simultaneously.* The entire body, each of its cells and systems, *all at the same time,* experiences 'the thought'. It is a magical and beautiful burst of activity happening all in the same *pico-second* throughout the entire body, synchronized fireworks exploding in all different areas at the same exact moment. But for all its beauty and humbling complexity, this sort of conclusion does nothing to help researchers trying to pinpoint the specific part of us that generates thought, our storehouse of consciousness.

It does, however, correlate precisely with the model of structured water, where water is constantly reforming and updating its structural information based on energetic principles and interactions. When the structural pattern of the water is altered, in an exacting and correct response to the energetic dynamics of any given situation situation, the physical systems that are operating within it immediately alter their structure or activity in response. The effect is immediate: all of the water in the body is operating as a part of one resonant information network system, and in fractions of an instant alters its structure, changing and updating its information. Consider the thought as the end result of an equation, or an algorithm. When energy travels among certain patterns and structure, the result of that equation will be a specific answer, i.e. a 'thought'. Our water structure can change every *trillionth and quadrillionth of a second* in order to update its information. When our energy travels among this new, changed, and updated information, the end result of that algorithm will again be a specific answer – one that is different from the first answer and equation, i.e. a different answer and thus a different 'thought.'

As we have seen, the structure of the water molecule has incredible impacts on electromagnetic frequencies, on protein structure and enzyme function, and brain stimulation. Once aware of water's properties, as well as its abundance and true functions in the physical body, it is easy to recognize how the entire body – the heart, the brain, the endocrine and immune system, and indeed every cell – can react *simultaneously* at the *instant* there is a conscious thought (actually the reaction is simultaneously in tandem the instant *before* we consciously register a 'thought'). Our consciousness is found in 99% of our molecules, stored in our complex network of liquid crystals and structured water, which also serves as the interface between our consciousness and our physical body.

Scientists calculate that the average person has 50,000-70,000 'thoughts' per day, and that anywhere from 90-98% of these will be the same thoughts as we had the day before. What we are seeing in these kinds of statistics are established patterns in our water molecules and the result of energy constantly cycling along these repeated patterns – causing our tendency towards repeated habits, repeated thoughts, and repeated ways of being, also called our personality and 'self'. This is how our consciousness expresses itself, or rather, *our* self, in and through our Water. The level of coherence in our body's water is determined by its level of structural integrity and complexity. We know that greater levels of coherence breed greater intelligence, self-value, and better quality of life, which translates into better decision making, expanded awareness and perception, and overall more positive thought patterns. Loss of structural integrity in our bio-waters causes reduced coherence, which breeds more negative thought patterns that in turn negatively affect the physical system and level of health. More positive thought patterns and greater coherence are also associated with having a greater sense of spirituality, as we see with people who regularly practice deep meditation. Later, as we explore sacred texts and the spiritual traditions and knowledge of structured water, we will understand why greater coherence in our water system could lead to a greater sense of spirituality.

An individual's consciousness and 'self' is a dynamic concept that is non-static and always changing. So how do we define it, in order to know what it is that is being stored in our water? It is widely held that while we are born as highly conscious beings, our experience of 'self' as an infant or newborn does not represent our developed consciousness. When one begins to complete the sentence "I am...(fill in the blank)", we do not refer to our 'Self' as what we represented in this infantile, or even childish, state. Rather, consciousness is often referred to as our experience of 'Self' through our collected thoughts, experiences, and memories. This implies an *evolution* of our consciousness, one that updates with new information and experiences, just like water. This evolution of our consciousness begins from the moment we experience self-awareness and memory, which begins at some point in-utero. Our Self as an infant *is* representative of our complete Self and individual consciousness, but it is more of a template, a framework, for what we will truly become as our collection of thoughts, experiences, and memories develop into what we would term our Self – our unique expression of consciousness.

As infants, we are often considered perfect, even holy, having not yet been scarred by the world and the experience of suffering. We are composed of *so much water,* and start the slow decline toward dehydration from day one. This water inside of us is *highly structured,* having (ideally) been exposed to little de-structuring energies as our bodies developed in the womb. Thus begins, from our primary experience as an "individual Self," the encoding of information and memory into our bio-water structures as we develop the brain function and compartmentalization methods to process this memory and information into our linear, language based thought patterns. Changes in our bio-energetic systems as we develop are also encoded into our bio-water, relaying to our physical form the state of the energetic systems, and cooperating in the physical manifestation and expression of the bio-energetics through bio-water's ability to interface with the physical systems and cellular networks, as we will explore in the next chapter.

So our water is not only critical in the storage of our memory and experiences, it is also representative of, and an active participant in, the *evolution* of our consciousness. Here we can begin to grasp the ultimate truth: *We Are Our Water,* a realization that comes full circle to the traditions of our cultural history and the truth our ancestors knew all along when they recognized *"water...as a reflection or an image of the Soul."* Our consciousness, what we term our Soul, or Spirit, our thoughts, memories, experiences, and perceptions of those experiences, emotions, beliefs, hopes, and regrets, are all reflected and encoded within the structure of our water. Our level of awareness, emotional and nonemotional reactions and perceptions, level of cognitive functioning, and focus and concentration, are determined by the structure of our bio-water. Our state of health, symptoms of disease, and physical functioning are all dependent upon the structure of the water in your body.

***You Are Your Water.***

# Chapter 16

# AN INTRODUCTION TO BIO-ENERGETICS

*Is it possible there exist human emanations that are still unknown to us? Do you remember how electrical currents and "unseen waves" were laughed at? The knowledge about humans is still in its infancy.*
~Einstein

We cannot take a real look at our body's structured water system, and thus be able to affect it for our benefit, without understanding its relationship to subtle energy. Subtle energy sciences are a very real branch of study, and it is helpful to have a background of knowledge in this area when examining how water works in the body to interface between the energies of consciousness and the energies of physical matter – even the energies of water itself as a physical 'substance'. For this reason, a brief introduction to subtle energy and bio-energetic systems is given here.

The realm of subtle energy has often been classified as "metaphysics", and as a result is sometimes quickly dismissed by mainstream science. With the introduction of energy healing practices such as Reiki in hospitals and clinical settings, and the number of scientific studies researching the effects of subtle energy, this is another outdated attitude that is rapidly changing. Subtle energy, or energy that is generally outside of our standard methods of perception and detection, is a very real form of energy, just as real as the electromagnetic frequencies we perceive. It is termed "subtle" because it is generally considered *less dense* than physical matter, but not any less real. The existence of subtle energy, also termed Chi, Prana, Vital Force, magneto-electricity, etc., in its various forms, has been demonstrated in countless traditions, experiments, observations, and research studies. We have already discussed a few researchers relating to water and healing energy or consciousness, which operate on the subtle energy spectrum, such as Drs. Vogel, Grad, Dean, Brame, and Schwartz. These researchers were and are all investigating the visible effects of invisible phenomena – the energies affecting water, individuals, and even vapors of gas – energies that clearly have effects and yet lay outside our methods of detection. This is the field of subtle energy, and it is a field that is growing everyday as new tools are developed, new phenomena recorded, and new studies undertaken.

The proof of the existence of subtle energy is undeniable and vast, and several competent and wonderful writers and researchers have undertaken the discussions around it. While these discussions are another area of study altogether and lay outside the scope of this book, we will suggest a few reference materials for more information on this subject which we highly recommend to anyone not already familiar and involved with it. Richard Gerber, M.D., has a fantastic book on subtle energy titled *Vibrational Medicine*, which discusses in easy terms the existence and basic fundamentals of the "multi-dimensional human anatomy", the energetic template of the human body and the bio-energetic systems which carry subtle energy and life force throughout the body.[1] These channels of subtle energy include the meridians of Traditional Chinese Medicine, a venous system for Chi and subtle energy, and the nadis of Ayurveda, which is the traditional Indian system of health and translates literally to *Science of Life*. These channels of subtle energy intersect at various points, creating a vortex of both outward energetic flow and inward energetic flow. In Traditional Chinese Medicine these are points used in acupuncture, in Ayurvedic medicine these are the Chakras, a Sanskrit word for *wheel*, and are also called 'marma points' (similar to acupuncture points).

In his book, Dr. Gerber cites many researchers and studies that support the existence of the realm of subtle energy. One such researcher is Dr. Kim Bong Han, who in the late 1960's found the physical meridian system – a very real venous-like system of ducts approximately 0.5-1.5 microns in diameter, which were found to carry extremely high concentrations of DNA, RNA, amino acids, free nucleotides, and various other essential hormones, including adrenaline and estrogen. This duct-like system, confirmed by more recent French studies, was found to form a vast and complex network throughout the body. Deep tubule systems were found along the surface of internal organs, throughout vascular and lymphatic vessels, the nervous system, and even within the layers of the skin. The duct system within the skin layers (referred to as the 'superficial system') corresponds to the meridians of classical acupuncture. The characteristics of the entire network – its direction of flow, entry and exit points through vessel walls, and

1. Gerber, Richard M.D. 2001.

the appearance of the larger physical systems developing *around* it, suggests that the meridian channels were formed prior to the physical development of the body, and perhaps even act as "spatial guides for the growth and development of the newly forming blood and lymphatic circulatory network."[2] Dr. Gerber also describes various studies exploring the effect of long distance healing, wherein subjects have been effective at manipulating vapors in chambers seemingly instantly, over incredible distances, and puts in understandable terms various studies involving healing, magnets, crystals, and other modalities operating on subtle energy.

Dr. Gerber is just one of many authors who has been reporting on these phenomena and the library of potential resources continue to grow. Dr. Gabriel Cousens's work, including *Spiritual Nutrition,* is a another potential resource, which like Dr. Gerber covers a variety of information and provides significant scientific evidence to support his position from a holistic M.D. perspective. For those looking for more technical descriptions of the physics behind this realm of energy, Dr. William Tiller's book *Science and Transformation* presents a well-modeled and founded theory for the existence of *magneto-electric energy,* as opposed to *electro-magnetic energy.* Dr. Tiller is a former professor in the department of Materials Science and Engineering at Stanford University, a former advisory physicist at Westinghouse Research Laboratories, has published over 275 scientific papers and three technical books, has been an associate editor for the Journal of Holistic Medicine, and is a founding director of both The Academy of Parapsychology and Medicine and The Institute of Noetic Sciences.

2. Gerber, Richard, M.D. 2001.

The term "magneto-electricity" coined by Dr. Tiller refers to a different spectrum of energy, or perhaps even an opposite polarity spectrum of energy, than that of our traditional electro-magnetic spectrum. In other words, it's either a polarity on the chart we have not yet recognized, or it's energy that's not on the chart at all. The traditional and current spectrum model displays only frequency bands with a higher ratio of electricity versus magnetism, which is why we call our perceivable energies *electromagnetic* rather than the other way around. Dr. Tiller proposes that those subtle energies which we cannot perceive and yet we know exist are more magnetic in nature, operating with a higher ratio of magnetism than electricity, and earning them the name *magneto-electric*. Tiller points to the similarities of structuring effects from water treated with magnetism versus water treated with healer's hands as one of the many supports for this theory, most of which are much more technical. The similarities between water structured by healers and water structured by magnets are astounding, and are not restricted to water alone – healer's hands have also been found to affect enzymes in a similar fashion to magnetic fields, they have in some instances have produced measurable magnetic fields from their hands themselves, and water treated by depressed patients displayed de-structuring and a reduction in enzyme activity. Tiller provides an in depth examination of the principles of magneto-electricity as determined by the observable effects of its influence, and he does so within a context of complex physics and geometric energetic lattices. These theories are perhaps the closest ones relating to structured energetics that this author has found, and one can see throughout Tiller's work the connection between the geometric energetic lattices and some of the underlying physics of the structure of energy throughout our Universe.[3]

> *We are dealing with storage phenomena of forces which are not in the electromagnetic area of the spectrum. Call it whatever you want... [if] you want to give them a name.*
> ~DR. MARCEL VOGEL
> SPEAKING ON ENERGIES AFFECTING
> THE STRUCTURE OF WATER

Whether we call it magneto-electricity, subtle energy, dark matter and dark energy ('dark' because we cannot see them, whether because of an absence of light or the presence of 'super-light' which is light that travels at 'faster than [visible] light speeds), or the 'cosmic microwave background', we are essentially talking about the energetics of consciousness and the fabric of our Universe, the underlying template and structure on which all things are built. These various terms (magneto-electricity, cosmic microwave background, dark matter/energy, subtle energy, Chi, Prana, etc.) may all relate to the same concept – those energies which play an essential role in the physical manifestation we experience around us, and are yet unseen – but these terms do not all share the same definition. Here, as we enter the realm of subtle energy within the body and physical systems, let us be clear that the subtle energy and bio-energetic systems are *not* the template and fabric of the structure of our space, but rather a form of manifested energy upon that plane, much in the way that we see manifested matter upon that plane.

Whether one is familiar with the reality of subtle

3. Tiller, William Ph.D. *Science and Human Transformation.* Walnut Creek, CA: Pavior Publishing, 1997.

energy or not does not change the fact that it does exist, and that the human body has its own subtle bio-energetic system, comprised of meridians (channels or vessels of subtle energy and bio-energetic matter), chakras, and the aura, which is the bio-energetic field surrounding all living organisms. In all likelihood the bio-energetic system is just as complex, if not more so, than our physical systems (of which we are still learning). Science has already confirmed much of the knowledge and theories passed to us from ancient cultures and traditions like Traditional Chinese Medicine and Ayurveda, who hand down a wealth of knowledge and study relating to the bio-energetic systems and connecting consciousness, energy, and health. While conventional Western medicine is the only health care system in the world that does not recognize the bio-energetic system, it will inevitably have to accept what science dictates: that our real physiological systems are based within our liquid crystal water system, where we see that the body truly is an incredible network of energy and information that is traveling through and conducted by geometric structures at incredible speeds, in incredibly complex environments.

Already we have developed diagnostic tools that enable us to recognize changes and disruptions in the way this energy and information is conducted through the body's subtle energetic systems, changes and disruptions that are precursors to physical manifestations of symptoms of disease. Disruptions in the energetic patterns and electromagnetic signatures of the liver, for example, are detectable weeks or even months prior to the development of physical symptoms. A variety of diagnostic tools have thus been created, mostly outside of the U.S., which typically rely on measuring electrical activity on the skin (called electro-dermal screening), stress testing, kinesiology (muscle testing), and biofeedback machines, to detect signs of dysfunction or disruptions within the energetic system of the body. Most often, these diagnostic tools are detecting energetic disturbances within the electromagnetic signatures and the energetic data that they register from the body. The body, and all of its components, emit electromagnetic frequencies, and certain devices have been developed which are capable of analyzing the recurring patterns within the electromagnetic frequencies, detecting disturbances or disharmonies within the pattern, and localizing them to a particular area or issue (i.e. the organ or system associated with that disturbance). Because the end-points of meridian lines on the skin (as used in acupuncture) exhibit very little electrical resistance, and have already been associated with the specific organs and tissues to which they relate through a system that has been tested and developed for over 5,000 years, meridian diagnostics through computerized instruments are one of the primary methods used by bio-energetic analysts. Once again the importance of patterns come into play, as preventative medicine through early diagnostics is finding its effectiveness by recognizing disturbances in the patterns of electromagnetic behavior, the perceivable aspect of our structured energy.

Another primary method of bio-energetic diagnostics is various forms of *bio-energetic photography*. Kirlian cameras, corona discharge mapping, and poly-interference photography have been developed in the market since the first Kirlian camera in 1939, and involve measuring or photographing the energy which radiates from all things, also called the corona discharge, gas discharge, electro-photonic 'glow' (i.e. 'energy light': electro=energy, photonic=light), or the aura. Today's advanced Kirlian photography systems include the Gas Discharge Visualization/Electro-photonic Capture (GDV/EPC) cameras, developed by Dr. Korotkov. GDV/EPC cameras have a reputed 98% accuracy in diagnostic assessments, and in 2000 were approved by the Ministry of Health in Russia as a permitted diagnostic technology in hospital and clinical settings. The GDV/EPC camera is just one of the several different forms of bio-energetic photography now available, which register the electromagnetic emanations of an individual (i.e. the 'aura') and translate it into a visual representation that we can see and analyze for disturbances in the patterns, density, and behavior of the bio-energetic system and the energetic field surrounding an individual. This type of analysis allows great insight into the functioning of the individual's bio-energetic system, allowing us to recognize and treat areas of disharmony and dysfunction before they manifest into physical symptoms. While a truly *preventative* medicine would attempt to prevent disruptions in the *energetic* system before they occur, these diagnostic developments, which allow us to prevent *physical* symptoms before they occur, are certainly the next best thing and are gaining momentum as a movement within the era of energetic medicine. As we continue to expand our understanding of the "multi-dimensional human anatomy", mankind becomes more aware of the true mechanics of their physical systems, through the lens of the modern technological era. And as more people become aware of the advantage and accuracy of such an approach to health, the resources dedicated to its development continue to increase exponentially.

# CHAPTER 17

# MANIFESTING ENERGETIC INFORMATION AT THE PHYSICAL LEVEL

*It followed from the special theory of relativity that mass [matter] and energy are both but different manifestations of the same thing – a somewhat unfamiliar conception for the average mind.*
~EINSTEIN

The most advanced scientific minds in human biology and medicine are those who have acknowledged the existence of the subtle bio-energetic system of the human body, and who conduct studies and investigation into developing a greater understanding of its system and how to better apply these fundamentals in our approach to health and wellness. These researchers have accepted the reality presented by our most ancient traditions concerning the body's subtle energy system, which is that our bio-energetic systems are manifesting information at the physical level, and have long sought the answer to *how* this phenomenon occurs. They continue to exert their efforts to discovering the mechanics driving the physical manifestation as a result of our bio-energetic systems, attempting to discover the precise method of action that relays disruptions in our subtle energy system to our physical bodies and as a result manifests symptoms of disease and disorder. This phenomenon is expressive of the complexity of the human body that has baffled men for centuries. This reality of our human anatomy, the tandem relationship between our bio-energetic systems and our physical body, is a result of our beautifully designed structured water system.

Our water system, with its incredible responsiveness to consciousness and energy, acts as an interface between our bio-energetic system and our physical expressions of biology and anatomy, translating subtle energy information into our physical expressions of structure, and thus health, wellness, and disease. Our bio-energetic systems are complex systems of subtle energy that exist, and persist, within our bodies. Already we know that disruptions in our bio-energetic systems manifest as physical symptoms of disease, and that this must occur through some type of interface that networks our subtle bio-energetic systems with our physical systems and the physical matter that comprises our biological processes. This interface occurs via the structure of the body's water, which not only reacts to changes in the bio-energetic system by adjusting its structure with new information, thereby affecting the development and expressions of our physical systems, but also by reacting to consciousness and other energies, through which it is able to incorporate structural changes that can affect *both* the physical system and the bio-energetic system. Our structured water system is truly the method of action in the feedback loop between our bodies, mind, and spirit.

This feedback loop between the loss of structure of the body's water and the manifestation and development of disease is no longer theory – pathologist Hoang Van Duc at the University of Southern California has successfully used a device known as a 'Magnetic Resonance Spectral Analyzer' (or MRA) to measure disruptions in cell waters to predict pre-pathological conditions – diseases that don't yet display any symptoms but which will develop into symptoms over time. When the water in the cellular fluids loses its structural integrity, it produces 'aberrant coherent information transfer', or irregular frequencies and changes in tissue resonance and vibration rates. By measuring the irregular shifts in frequency using the MRA, "pre-pathological conditions have been predicted, detected, and later confirmed based upon aberrant shifts in tissue resonance."[1]

It may seem like a lot to take in, but consider what we have already learned. The structural integrity and energetic capacities of DNA are dependent upon the geometric complexity of the water that surrounds it. The life of the cell and its ability to receive, decode, and transmit the electromagnetic frequencies that are necessary for proper biological processes is dependent upon the geometric complexity of the water that is within and surrounding the cell. The level of hydration necessary for optimum health is dependent upon the geometric complexity of the water in the body. A loss of structural integrity, or a change in structural patterns, affects the health of the DNA, the cell, and the hydration levels in the body, which in turn manifest as physical symptoms of disease and disorder. Thus we see that as these physical symptoms are preempted by changes in the bio-energetic systems, these bio-energetic systems must be affecting the structure of the bio-waters.

The feedback loop between our bio-energetic systems,

---

1. Cherniske, Stephen. *Aqua Resonance.*

our bio-water systems, our consciousness experience, and our physical systems is complex and centered around the bio-water interface. Any incoming energy and information to our bodies, including subtle energy, affects the structure of our bio-waters and therefore has an effect on our bio-energetic and physical systems. As we already discussed, the structure of our bio-waters is also intimately connected to our experience of thought patterns and our current state of consciousness, and as a result, our feedback loop looks something like this: the structure of our waters determines our consciousness and physical state, its level of structure and coherence is directly responsible for our thought patterns and our physical function. In turn, the state of our thought patterns affects the level of structure and coherence of our waters, which loops back and reflects this in our thought patterns and physical health. When our waters lack certain geometric coherence, we experience negative thought patterns, which in turn contribute to more de-structuring of our waters, and this growing entropic structure thus continues to feed the cycle of negative thought patterns.

The traditional model of our biofeedback loop emphasizes making changes in the consciousness of the mind in order to change the energetic and physical systems of the body. Because of the dynamics of the mind-body-spirit relationship this is effective, but is extremely challenging for most people. Making changes in the consciousness and the mind in order to have true changes in our ways of being, ways of perceiving, and ways of living is something that people find incredibly difficult. We call our habits 'ingrained', and often times people find themselves unable to truly make such changes until they hit a 'rock-bottom' which may or may not mean facing their own mortality. Habits that are 'ingrained' are nothing more than established patterns, which yes, can be changed by making conscious choices and 'thinking differently'. But it is our level of consciousness and our habitual ways of thinking that got us here in the first place, driving our behavior and the choices we make at that level. In pointing first to making changes in our mind and consciousness, we assume that we can change our behavior and choices from the same level of consciousness that drives the ones we want to change, and assume that we can raise to a different level of consciousness and experience different thought patterns even though our 'system', our current level of consciousness, is only capable of reflecting and computing itself, the level it is on. What proponents of the mind-body-spirit approach are missing, and in fact what everyone has failed to recognize, is that the mind, body, and spirit are all sitting on our template of *water*. When we look at ourselves, our beings of water, what reflects back at us is our body, mind, and spirit. We are merely reflections of our water's crystallography, and subject to its driving forces – determining our thoughts, and defining our perceptions and experiences, our bodies, minds, and spirits.

But by stepping forward into this bio-feedback loop, we recognize a greater opportunity for efficient and positive effect: by raising the structure of our bio-waters, increasing its complexity, fractality, and coherence, we will effectively change what it reflects and manifests – our mind, our experience of spirit, and our physical bodies. By raising the structure of our bio-waters, we can improve our bio-energetic system (and thus our physical health), and drive greater states of coherency and consciousness that lead to an improved quality and experience of life, as well as greater longevity and wellness. In looking at what drives the mind-body-spirit connection, we see deeper into ourselves to recognize what it is that is manifesting and directing that system. No longer must our experience be unwittingly subject to our level of crystallography – instead, we can apply this knowledge to affect our level of crystallography in order to change our experience, our thought patterns, our habits, and ourselves. Our bio-waters rapidly react to new information and structure in response, affecting both the bio-energetic and physical systems. If we can understand how to achieve an increase in the structural complexity, integrity, and flexibility of our bio-waters, we could become successful in helping to *determine* the results of our bio-feedback loop, rather than being at its mercy.

# PART IV

# SACRED WATER, STRUCTURED WATER

*Science without Spirituality is Lame.*
~EINSTEIN

*The true foundation of all culture is the knowledge and understanding of Water.*
~VIKTOR SCHAUBERGER

To truly understand what water is, we must reach outside the limitations and boxes of mainstream, or even unconventional, science. We must reach into our own cultural history, the relationship humanity has had with water throughout antiquity, and what the wisdom of ancient texts and the documents of the sages and the saints tell us about water. When we combine what we know about water from a scientific standpoint with what we know about water from our spiritual roots, we find the way to a more complete understanding.

*In many cases [of cultural history], water
appears as a reflection or an image of the Soul.*
~DR. CHRISTOPHER WITCOMBE
PROFESSOR OF ART HISTORY

Let us examine the above quote, from a Boston
University professor of Art History. "In many cases, water
appears as a reflection or an image of the Soul." Looking
at what we know about water's structuring capacity and
its ability to reflect the information of consciousness, and
the information of *our* consciousness, within its
molecular arrangement, we see that the cultural historical
perspective of water as a reflection of the Soul is a more
accurate description than we may have ever before
realized. Believing that all ancient knowledge and
cultural perspectives prior to the modern era were
strictly metaphors severely cripples the meaning we can
extrapolate and gain from their teachings. The structure
of water truly *does* reflect consciousness, and when water
has stored the information from the consciousness of an
individual – as does the water in our bodies – considering
it as an image of the Soul may be more apt than we ever
realized. And since Water does not just store the
information of *individual* consciousness, but **all
consciousness and energy information,** Water becomes
not only an image of the Soul but also an image of energy,
consciousness, and the Creator. Recognized as such, the
reverence for water held by ancient peoples expressed
itself in a variety of practices, traditions, and teachings.
Every major religion and nearly *all* ancient traditions,
from Hinduism, Judeo-Christianity, and Islam, to
Egyptian, Greek, and Babylonian mythology, recognize
that the birth of life arose from Water, and that there the
spark of Life, the spirit of God, and the essence of the All,

abides or can be found within it. It is believed to purify the soul, cleanse the spirit, remove energetic impurities, and wash away sin and karma. We find evidence of this in healing springs and bathing rituals, in 'water-priestess' clan titles, in water preachers and baptism rituals. It expresses itself in countless texts, scriptures, survived legends, and verbal traditions. Literature from ancient India, Egyptian mythology, the Bible, the Torah, the Qur'an, un-canonized apocrypha work and gnostic scriptures, all describe a holy essence of Water. By examining even a few of these texts and practices, we find descriptions of the amazing abilities of water's remarkable structure and our ancestral explanation for what this structure truly means. It would appear these various traditions were all operating on principles of structured water science, within a model of structured water consciousness that intimately connects our mind, consciousness, and spirit with the structure of our water. These examinations also reveal a deep connection between structured water consciousness and enlightenment, spiritual evolution, and everlasting eternal life – teachings from which we can gain much understanding.

*Once we have reached the level of geometry, form, and structure, we are at the level of the spirit, or rather the manifestation of the spirit into matter.*
~DR. MARCEL VOGEL

CHAPTER 18

# SACRED SPRINGS, HEALING
# WATERS

*The apostle...who dwelt at the city of Jerusalem; a healer whose
medicine was Water, a healer that healeth....(that) which go forth... to
destroy the physical body... Then Yahia-Yuhana took the
Jordan [waters from the River Jordan] and the medicine Water... and
he cleansed lepers, opened the eyes of the blind, and lifted the broken
(maimed) to walk on their feet...*
~ FRAGMENTS OF MANDAEAN SCRIPTURE

Through understanding the science of water and its
connection to health, healing, disease, and longevity, we
can gain a new appreciation for the wisdom of our
ancestral traditions in the concept of 'healing water', 'holy
water', and 'sacred water'. For thousands of years, certain
waters have been known to help cure illness and have
miraculous restorative and spiritual powers. These sacred
waters, revered by virtually every culture, are usually
connected with significant or miraculous events and are
highly structured (or were, as the case may be in certain
now polluted areas). It is their high structure that lends
them properties different from ordinary water, a fact
recognized by many peoples and the responsible factor
for the overwhelming anecdotal evidence of healing

experiences. In fact, prior to modern history it was well-established knowledge that certain waters had these amazing properties, thus they were referred to as 'holy', 'healing', 'sacred', or 'living'. This is the pre-modern science understanding, where the physical changes in properties of the water was not the focus of the people, but the actual event of physical and spiritual healing. It was not a phenomena to investigate, it was a phenomena to live and experience, and the respect and regard for the Water likely played a large part in the individual's connection to the Water consciously, not influencing it and degrading its structure with doubt or negative belief but rather reinforcing the positive structure through their acceptance and knowingness of the Water's power.

References to various sacred springs, pools, and other healing water sites occur at the beginning of human history, and the use of sacred Water is one of mankind's oldest religious traditions. Healing waters and baths also find great appreciation in the world's oldest medical literature, with the extensive writings by Hippocrates, the 'father of modern medicine', over 2,500 years ago detailing the healing of diseases with water. Today, at the foot of the Temple Mount in Jerusalem, one can still see beside the stairs where the Levites would be arranged in welcoming choirs next to the remains of the stone ritual baths used for the spiritual preparation of pilgrims. Before the revelation of Moses at Mount Sinai, the peoples assembled at the base of the mountain were commanded to immerse themselves in preparation for coming face to face with God. In England, we find hundreds of known sacred water sites, with over 100 'holy wells' in Cornwall alone. People still flock to the waters at St. Bernard's well in Stockbridge, St. Brigid's well in Ireland, St. Inan's well in Scotland, the Su

Tempiesu well in Italy, the Chalice Well at Glastonbury, and the holy well at Chartres in France, just to name a few, for their curative and healing powers. These curative powers have no restraint, and the stories told by those who witness or experience it say it is capable of curing everything from blindness, to paralysis, arthritis, broken bones, skin conditions, and even mental illness.

Although many of the water sites just mentioned are areas attributed to Christian saints, most were already sacred long before the birth of Christianity. The Celts honored certain wells and natural springs for their medicinal and sacred values, and many of these were renamed by the Church to assist the transition from 'paganism' to Christianity by rededicating the water to a saint. The tradition of holy wells, alive and thriving during Celtic and Druidic times, slowly devolved over generations to be replaced by the practice of wishing wells and other tales. Meanwhile mineral baths and hot spring baths, known to effect cures for a variety of diseases and ailments, have remained widely popular across the world, and are renowned for being places of pilgrimage and healing. The mineral springs at Bath in England have been in use for at least 7,000 years, and even more famous are the rituals of the great Roman, Greek, Russian, Finnish, or Turkish Baths. These groups spent great effort and architecture in developing beautiful and functional bathhouses for the people, which were originally intended for healing, curative, and therapeutic purposes. Some of Rome's greatest architecture is their bathhouses, which at one point numbered nearly 1,000 in the city alone.[1] When the focus in some areas began to shift from one of healing to one of social gathering, the

---

1. Ebner, Kevin. *Health and Healing through Water.* University of Oregon: Scholars Bank.

influx of conservative religious perceptions issued taboos on all bathhouses as being immodest and advocated private bathing. Consequently, the dedication to *hydrotherapy*, or water therapy and water cures, has largely become a lost tradition over recent centuries. Today we unknowingly see it in the acronym 'Spa' (i.e. spa tub, resort spa), which stands for the term 'solus par aqua', literally meaning 'health or healing through water'. These are just a few examples of our historical relationship with the concept of 'healing water', which clearly has held its place throughout time in the abundance of sacred springs, rivers, baths, and lakes, and the countless traditions and accounts of the miraculous healings, cures, and therapies associated with them.

> *Now there is in Jerusalem by the Sheep Gate a pool, which is called in Hebrew Bethesda, having five porches. In these lay a great multitude of sick people, blind, lame, paralyzed, waiting for the moving of the water.*
> *For an angel went down at a certain time into the pool and stirred up the water, then whoever stepped in first, after the stirring of the water, was made well of whatever disease he had.*
> ~BIBLE, NEW TESTAMENT: JOHN 5:2-4

The above description by St. John of miraculous water healings is one echoed by cultures across time and region. The use of healing springs and wells is still very much alive today, though not as common as it once was prior to industrialization, pollution, and the rise of the stiff-necked science systems that dominate Europe and Western thought, which have a tendency to deny or ignore that which they cannot explain or mathematically calculate. There are many recently discovered famous healing waters, in addition to the time-honored holy sites, and all come with their own remarkable and similar testimonies. In Germany, east of Dusseldorf, a newly discovered healing spring in an abandoned slate mine cave is reported to have cured a woman of blindness, fixed an ex-miner's crippling back pain, and regulated and stabilized a woman with high blood pressure. In 2006 a Switzerland spring at the home of a group of Franciscan nuns was reported to have healing effects, as was the spring at the Benedictine monastery near Zurich, a mountain spring in the Alps near eastern Switzerland, and a spring in central Switzerland at the birthplace of Bruder Klaus, the 15th century hermit revered as the 'father of Swiss neutrality'. In 2007, an abandoned, formerly fouled and rubbish filled well in Pasir Putih, Malaysia, began gushing crystal clear and 'sweet smelling' water, reputed by the locals and those who pilgrimage to the site to have healing powers.[2]

In 2005 in southern Philippines, a fountain of water was discovered to produce water less than a foot from the surface, remarkable for the surrounding area where ground water can only be extracted from deep underground. A man walking past the water coming up from the dry ground drank some and applied it to his arthritic elbow, and moments later the pain was gone. News of its curative effects spread rapidly throughout the region, and today thousands of people have visited the site, including a 70 year old woman interviewed by the local paper, who described herself as suffering severe back pain and bent posture prior to being rubbed down with the wet soil. After she was wiped clean with the water from the fountain, she attests that her pain has

2. Ariff, S. "Miracle water from murky well." *New Straits Times*. 10 Nov. 2007: Malaysia.

subsided and she can now stand and walk straight.[3] The stories continue to accumulate as more and more people make the pilgrimage and apply the power of sacred healing waters in their life.

Healing waters on the grounds of Mount St. Mary's College in Maryland, the oldest Mary shrine in the United States, has reportedly cured deafness, tuberculosis, and a variety of other ailments. Vermont is also home to several famous healing springs sites, as is California, both with their associated testimonies of healings and curative powers. In Australia, seven adjoining sheep and cattle farms attribute their livestock's longer lifespans, greater fertility, and better health (as compared to neighboring livestock) to the healing spring from which the animals drink. A healing spring at the Wang Kanai Temple in Thailand is reputed to have miraculous healing effects and cure many life-threatening, painful, and debilitating conditions, including five paralyzed people who reportedly now walk unaided.

In Tlacote, Mexico, after the water from a local well was witnessed healing the owner's dog, he began giving the water away – to hundreds and thousands of people who come from all over the world, said to sometimes draw more than 10,000 in a single day. It is reported to have cured AIDS, cancer, diabetes, and numerous other ailments. Thus, Tlacote has been nicknamed 'The Mexican Lourdes,' referencing the most famous healing waters of all still recognized today. While the ranch at Tlacote has closed since the death of its owner, it is still held as one of the most well known healing water sites, even drawing attention from celebrities like Magic Johnson. The research that has been done on the Tlacote

3. "Mindanao is Holy Ground." *Asian Journal.* 22 Jul 2011: San Diego, CA.

waters indicate that it weighs less than normal water and contains six additional crystalline compounds, as well as trace minerals. A professor at the Graduate School of Genetic Resources and Technology is reputed to have also found an unusually high concentration of atomic hydrogen, perhaps accounting for its lighter weight. Still, none of the variances in composition are found to account for the miraculous healings associated with the waters at Tlacote.

The Lourdes of France that Tlacote is nicknamed after is one of the most famous healing water sites in the world, drawing *six million people every year* to a town of 15,000. It is home of the site where St. Bernadette Soubirous received visions of the Virgin Mary, who instructed Bernadette to drink from the spring in the grotto of Massabielle, in Lourdes. Shortly after, people began to make pilgrimages to the site and miraculous healings began to be recorded. The water has been channeled to flow into a 450,000-liter reservoir that feeds many small fountains, allowing hundreds of people to immerse themselves daily in Lourdes water. Nearly 7,000 unexplained healings have been *recorded*, which represent a small percentage of the actual healing events experienced at the site. In order to ensure the claims of cures, Pope Saint Pius X requested the establishment of the Lourdes Medical Bureau, which rigorously investigates claims of miraculous healing. Of the 7,000 people that have reported their case as a miracle, the Bureau has declared 68 cases as scientifically inexplicable miracles. As part of their intense scrutiny, the Bureau allows all qualified medical doctors to have unlimited access to the files and documents at the Bureau, allowing them to conduct their own critical investigations. In the majority of the vast number of cases, the medical

authorities upheld the event as beyond medical
explanation. Lourdes water has been found to have higher
oxygen levels, as well as concentrations of Germanium,
which account for some, but not all, of its properties, and
otherwise appears to be fairly standard spring water –
traces of minerals, while overall relatively pure and inert.
Neither the trace minerals, level of purity, high oxygen
levels, or the inclusion of germanium accounts for the
healings or other observations of Lourdes water
properties. The strong and consistent effect that small
amounts of Lourdes water added to other water samples
has on the pH of the water samples is a phenomenon that
is not accounted for by any of the chemical constituents
in the water itself – and there is no scientific explanation
for why a small amount of Lourdes water would balance
and/or alkalize other water samples. Similar effects have
been noted with chlorine, wherein small amounts of
Lourdes water is added to samples containing free
chlorine, and as a result we can observe a breakdown in
the chlorine, and a slowing of the chlorine concentration
levels.[4]

Among all the revered water sites, the Ganga River is
regarded as particularly sacred, and is our planet's most
famous holy water site. Among the Hindu and Vedic
cultures, the Ganga is the most spiritually powerful and
potent body of water on Earth. Its energetic source of
manifestation is believed to be the pure water of the
Divine Ocean, and it is said to come from the lotus feet
of God before descending onto the planet. Manifesting
in the Himalayas, the 'rooftop of the world' and the
'mountains of the gods', it descends to the plains of India
as if from Heaven. This sentiment resonates strongly with

4. Ansaloni A. *Effect of Lourdes water on water pH*. Boll Chim Farm. 2002 Jan-
Feb;141(1):80-3.

the Ancient Egyptian's feelings regarding the Nile, which they taught also descended from the house of Heaven and manifested as the river which flowed to the Egyptian plains. Bathing in its waters is believed to cleanse away karma and cause the remission or removal of sins, called 'papa' in Sanskrit, a term used to describe the actions that create negative karma by violating moral and ethical codes, which brings negative consequences – i.e. sin and its consequences. It is through this quality that it also is believed to facilitate the 'liberation from the cycle of life and death,' capable of cleansing lifetimes of karma so that one may reach ascension to Nirvana (Heaven). In these traditions, a full cleansing of karma allows one to ascend to heaven, not having to re-incarnate to once again experience the suffering of life, stuck in a karmic wheel of life and death from accumulated karma.

The River Ganges is so revered that it is home to the largest gathering on Earth, which occurs in India during the holy time of Kumbh Mela, a sacred time lasting 55 days and recurring every 12 years, a time that has been celebrated for centuries throughout the Hindu and Vedic traditions. In February of 2013, over 50 million people immersed themselves in the waters of the Ganga during this holy festival, which coincided during this time to a unique planetary alignment that occurs once every 147 years, making it particularly auspicious for those who made the pilgrimage. For most non-believers, this sort of practice seems at the very least merely symbolic in nature, if not completely ludicrous – consider a town of 1.2 million people swelling to host the over 100 million bathers, and then sharing with them that same water. And while the principles of 'washing away sin' or 'cleansing karma' will be examined later, let us here simply begin by opening ourselves up to the connections between sacred healing waters and structured water science.

The water of the River Ganges has unique properties and qualities, in spite of the strain it suffers from high levels of pollution. It is reputed to have 25 times higher dissolved oxygen levels than normal rivers, aiding in its ability to handle the biochemical oxygen demand levels it requires to keep a certain level of purification, and allowing the waters to clean suspended wastes 15 to 20 times faster than other rivers.[5] Because of this, it exhibits a wonderful self-purification and anti-putrification quality (wherein the water stays fresh and does not putrefy, water putrefies as a result from the growth of anaerobic bacteria which leaves that stale water smell). The Malaria Research Center in New Delhi has observed that water from the upper reaches of the Ganga did not host mosquito breeding, and also appeared to prevent mosquito breeding in other waters it was added to. British physician E. Hanbury Hankin reported in the French journal *Annales de l'Institut Pasteur* the death of the deadly cholera bacterium within three hours of exposure to waters of the River Ganges. The same bacteria tested in distilled water were observed still thriving 48 hours later.[6]

These remarkable qualities of the Ganga are attributed to two primary factors: the presence of *bacteriophages* (viruses which kill bacteria, i.e. anti-bacterial properties) and an "unknown factor, which gives it the unusual ability to retain higher amounts of dissolved oxygen from the atmosphere".[7] By now we recognize these properties

5. Bhargava, D.S. Benthasludge Stabilization in the River Ganga at Kanpur. *Indian Journal of Environmental Protection.* Jan 10, 2011.
6. Kalshian, Rakesh. Ganges Has Magical Cleaning Properties. *Geographic* 66:5. April 1994.

as an expression of the water's specific structure, one that works in tandem with the belief and consciousness of the people and its experience of the environment. The water of the Ganga, in its high responsiveness to consciousness as a structured liquid crystal, and as a revered, respected, honored, and worshipped water source by hundreds of millions of people, is able to maintain a level of structure capable of expressing the properties we have thus described, although the recent exponential rise in pollution is having a negative effect on the biochemical oxygen demand levels, and is thus degrading the natural self-purifying abilities of the Ganga.

While the River Ganges is known for its spiritual purification and cleansing power, we also know that water can be structured specifically to endow it with anti-bacterial and cleansing properties. In Japan and Korea, scientists have been raising the pH level of water from a 7 to a 9.2 on the acid scale by exposing water to various magnets and electromagnetic fields.[8] This type of structural change so dramatically affects the property of water that it increases its dissolving and caustic power, antiseptic qualities, and antioxidant potential – making it an excellent cleansing agent. Clearly, a high cleansing ability is certainly a quality of specifically structured water, as are its healing potentials. Already we have examined the necessary role that structured water plays in our body and with our DNA, and have seen that diseases are associated with poorly structured cellular water and a loss of structure in the water surrounding the

7. Mukherjee, D., Chattopadhyay, M., Lahiri, S.C. Water Quality of the River Ganga (The Ganges) and Some of its Physico-Chemical Properties. *The Environmentalist*. 13:3, 199-210. 1993.
8. Lam, Michael M.D. Magnetized Water. Body Mind Nutrition. 2001. Web. Accessed June 2013.

DNA. Since we also know that cancer cells do not and cannot exist in highly structured water, the cleansing and purifying aspects of the Ganga and other renowned water sites are of course not limited to spiritual purification, but actual physical cleansing and healing properties.

This is not surprising, as the groups that follow the spiritual water purification – which include those whose practice Islam, Hindu, Vedas, Gnosticism, Judaism, and Christianity – usually believe that diseases, afflictions, and ailments are usually a product of karma and/or sin, either acquired in the current lifetime or previous lives. While the concept of sin carrying through over various reincarnations is not discussed in Judeo-Christian literature, it is well established among the Hindu and Vedic traditions, and several others. In these traditions, the general concept is that sin is accumulated and carried over through the reincarnated lifetimes of an individual soul, and thus affects the experience of the individual in this lifetime through the laws of cause and effect – as accumulated sin brings negative consequences, or hardships, which create the opportunity for either the clearing of sin through positive action, or the accumulation of more sin through negative response. This process is the method of the soulful evolution or de-evolution in the experience of the individual, with total soulful evolution (associated with enlightenment, ascension, and heaven) being the ultimate goal, in order to release one from continuing to suffer the karmic cycle of life and death in the material and physical world. The material and physical world is also referred to as *the illusion* in many traditions, lending support to the quantum physics and consciousness models wherein the physical reality is an illusion comprised of consciously manifested energy – thus our physical reality only *appears* real while really being manifested energy, or light. It is interesting to note that while mainstream Judeo-Christians do not discuss accumulated sin in regards to reincarnated individual experiences, they do refer to one being subject to and carrying the 'sins of their fathers', which expresses multiple meanings, some of the most common interpretations are as metaphor referencing the handing down of genetic flaws (or sin stored within the genome of the male parent), or referring to how an individual is, at some level, a product of their parents and their parenting.

Reincarnation itself however, *is* recognized in Judeo-Christian traditions (as well as Islam and Hinduism). It was said, for example, that Jesus would reincarnate in physical form, and that Elijah would return – later we learn that Elijah had returned (or reincarnated) as John the Baptist, through the direct words of Jesus. A primary figure in Christianity, John the Baptist is well known for his practice and preaching of water rituals for the cleansing of sin and spiritual purification. He was chosen to perform the water baptism of Jesus, who also promoted baptism and water purification. Both of these figures, along with all of the world's major religions and countless minor ones, were in many ways various forms of what we could call 'water preachers' for their emphasis on the powers, traditions, and uses of Water.

In any event, it is certainly interesting that the same waters used for *spiritual and religious purification* are known for having *healing and curative properties*, as well as properties of *material and bacterial cleansing*. These 'sacred waters' are highly structured, and highly structured water is a stronger solvent, more absorbent, and antibacterial, and, in following the law of 'as above, so below (and everywhere in between)', it makes sense that the structural abilities of water which make it capable of cleansing and purifying material substances and healing physical illnesses would also be capable of purifying the spirit, energy, and consciousness of an individual, and clearing them of sin and karma. In this instance sin and karma can be thought of as the energetic waste, dirt, or tarnish on the soul, spirit, or energy body of an individual, washed clean by highly structured water. In this way, we see a connection between energetic and physical principles, where (structured) water's physical properties of healing and cleansing are emblematic of its corresponding energetic properties of healing and cleansing. This principle, that of spiritual and consciousness purification and cleansing through Water, absolutely permeates nearly *every* religious tradition – so much so that once examined, all of these traditions appear at their core to be 'water-based religions'.

# CHAPTER 19

# WATER PREACHERS

---

*Jesus answered, Truly, truly, I say to you, except a man be born of water and of the Spirit, he cannot enter into the kingdom of God.*
~BIBLE, NEW TESTAMENT: JOHN 3:5

Throughout history, people have not just revered Water and its healing and spiritual purification properties, they have seen it as a focal point and foundation of their religious traditions. All of the world's major religions: Hinduism, Islam, Christianity, and Judaism, as well as countless minor religions – African, Egyptian, South American, and Asian traditions, Gnosticism, and Vedic traditions (similar to Hinduism), for example – all express a foundation of structured water principles, practices, and teachings within their respective traditions. Any group that ascribes the way to attain Heaven, enlightenment, Christ, purity, perfection, eternal life, or the cleansing of sin or spiritual impurities through any form of water or baptismal practice can essentially be called a 'water-preacher' – one who is preaching a way to Heaven, God, or spiritual purity through the power of Water. Although not always recognized, all of these

traditions attest to these principles, albeit sometimes
indirectly.

While the focus of 'salvation' or 'spiritual
enlightenment' is discussed in many terms, evaluating
some of the various beliefs of water and spiritual purity
reveals a fundamental pervasive understanding of the
attainment of spiritual purity being based in water rituals.
The Vedic and Hindu practices with the River Ganges,
Christian and Gnostic baptism rituals, Hebrew water
rituals and *mikvahs* (sacred water cleansing baths), the
water purification rituals of Buddhism and other Asian
spiritual groups, and the Islamic practice of *ghusl* and
*wudu* (washing before prayer in ritually pure water) are
obvious expressions of some of these water-based beliefs.
It is a pervasive theme throughout human antiquity, and
to explore the many traditions of the world and their
respective structured water beliefs and practices would
be a massive undertaking and potentially volumes of
work. Here, we will simply explore some examples of
different beliefs and traditions from a variety of time
periods and locations, as we have already done with
several healing water sites. These traditions involve not
only water rituals, structuring practices, and spiritual
purification methods, but also mysterious ancient
structures and their intimate connection with structured
water.

The Great Pyramid of Giza is perhaps the most
mysterious and hotly debated structure on our planet,
as well as the largest and most accurately constructed
building in the world. And while it may come as a
surprise, it is also deeply connected with ancient water
rituals and structuring methods. For years the
controversy has raged on regarding who was responsible
for the Great Pyramid's construction, how they were able

to accomplish such a remarkable feat, and when such a marvel was actually erected. The answers provided by mainstream Egyptology do not hold up under examination. There is mounting geological evidence that dates the Great Pyramid much earlier than even pre-dynastic Egypt, and indisputable weathering patterns on the Sphinx which date it even older than the Pyramid itself, and which indicate the Sphinx was erected at least 10,000 years ago. Mainstream Egyptology or even mainstream history cannot accept this evidence, which contradicts all of our belief of the 'primitive' abilities of our ancestors 10,000 years ago and pre-dynastic Egypt. Instead they have made a calculated decision in refusing an earlier dating on these epic structures, which are magnificent, unexplainable, and irreproducible feats of architecture. Wanting to maintain that progress must happen in a linear fashion, mainstream Egyptology insists that the hundreds of sub-standard pyramids located in Egypt must have been made first, and the building practices must have developed and improved over time until they were able to accomplish the Great Pyramid. To imply otherwise is to say that ancient Egyptians actually *regressed* in knowledge and progress, rather than advancing it, going from whoever was responsible for the building of the Great Pyramid and the Sphinx and regressing in knowledge and capabilities to whoever was responsible for the Step Pyramid and the hundreds of failed and deteriorating pyramids, built using an entirely different method of construction. Evidence continues to accumulate for the Great Pyramid's construction occurring *prior* to the smaller, poorly constructed pyramids. The Pyramids at Giza give no indication of being related to tomb use in any way (there is no evidence anywhere of anyone ever being buried in the Pyramids of Giza), nor do these ancient Pyramids contain reliable inscriptions or hieroglyphs of any kind (except those which came much later than its original construction). So what were the original Giza Pyramids for?

Outside of official Egyptology, the theories regarding the Pyramid's purpose and builders are quite diverse and range in plausibility – from acoustic levitation building practices, to being constructed by ancient aliens, or for serving as some kind of spiritual initiation temple for pre-Ancient Egyptians. Most of these theories are quite outlandish, and few hold little, if any, water. The most promising theory answering the question of *how* the Great Pyramid was constructed comes from French architect Jean-Pierre Houdin, and involves the use of an interior ramp. The most promising theory regarding its *purpose* has been proposed by Edward Kunkel in 1965, and further refined by John Cadman, Edward Malkowski, and others. Their work examines the relationship between the construction of the Great Pyramid and its associated *subterranean aquifer and aqueduct system* (underground water system). They provide a testable theory using scientific experimentation that takes into account *all* of the architectural features of the Great Pyramid – including the mysterious 'Queen' and 'King's Chambers', the 'Great Gallery' (a 153 ft. long, 29 ft. high, and 7 ft. wide passage way), and the use of granite stones lining the Grand Gallery, as well as in and above the chambers themselves.[1] Their work demonstrates that the Great Pyramid actually functioned to structure water, to pump and channel structured water to available areas for access and agriculture, and to use the energy generated by the hydraulic system of the Great Pyramid to generate

1. Malkowski, Edward. *Ancient Egypt 39,000 BCE: The History, Technology, and Philosophy of Civilization X.* Vermont: Bear & Co. 2010.

pulsed extremely low-frequency (ELF) electromagnetic energy across the region (similar to the Schumann Resonance or natural Earth frequency).

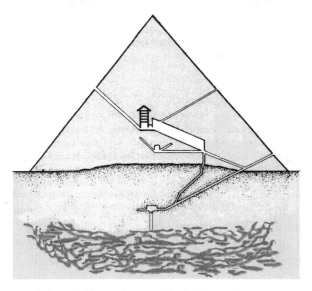

Fig. 13: Great Pyramid of Giza diagram,
with subterranean aquifer.

The research was extensive, and involved working models using the layout and schematics of the Great Pyramid's design, including the subterranean aquifer, the subterranean chamber, and its associated tunnels. The subterranean chamber is about 46 feet long by 28 feet wide (or 14 by 8.5 meters), and is located 100 feet below ground in the exact center of the pyramid, 586 feet beneath the apex tip of the pyramid. Attached to it are a series of branching tunnels, connecting to the old location of the Nile River (which has migrated east several miles over the past thousands of years, but at one point was much closer to the Giza Plateau and the Great

Pyramid). The water from the Nile and the subterranean aquifer provided the water source for the structuring and pumping action of the Great Pyramid. The working model Cadman created using the design of the Great Pyramid's construction operated as an effective water pump, creating a whirlpool of vortexing water in a square pit that is carved into the subterranean chamber. Additionally, he found that the action of the pump (when embedded underground, as it was embedded in the limestone bedrock in the real subterranean chamber) created a *vertical compression wave*, a sort of periodic vibration or shock wave. By adjusting the back pressure one can change the water's density, altering the compression wave's velocity and frequency and allowing for a sort of 'fine tuning' of the Great Pyramid's standing wave generation. The standing compression wave emanating from the subterranean chamber was transformed into acoustic sound as it traveled up the pyramid, causing the granite to resonate, vibrate, or 'sing', projecting its sound into the atmosphere and creating an electromagnetic field in the surrounding area.[2] The subtle electrical field created by the Great Pyramid would essentially create a canopy to deflect 'very low frequency' (VLF) and 'extremely low frequency' (ELF) energy into the surrounding area, electromagnetic frequencies that are essential for Life, promote health, and improve plant growth. Thus, the Great Pyramid functioned not just as a water pump, but also as a structuring unit – using the power of movement, vortexing, and acoustic and standing wave elements to affect the quality of the water, which was then distributed for use by the surrounding areas. It also functioned as an ELF generator,

2. Malkowski, Edward. *Ancient Egypt 39,000 BCE: The History, Technology, and Philosophy of Civilization X.* Vermont: Bear & Co. 2010.

broadcasting beneficial extremely low frequencies into the environment. This is, of course, a *very* brief and simplified version of this explanation, which has been thoroughly detailed and engineered by Cadman and others. And while we may never truly know the beliefs and traditions of the culture that created the Ancient Pyramids, whoever they may be, we can assume from their advanced knowledge of hydraulics, acoustics, and structured water principles that they are our oldest known civilization of water-preachers. These pre-Ancient Egyptians would have preached principles of water and structuring techniques, as well as beneficial and highly structuring frequency generation and application, with their use of pulsed extremely low-frequency electromagnetic energy radiations and structuring methods to assist plant growth, agriculture, and health.

Another great mystery of human history is the famous Nazca Lines of the Nazca Valley in Peru. Like the Great Pyramid, the purpose of the Nazca Lines were hotly debated since their discovery, but have since been connected to the ancient understanding held by the Nazca people regarding water, particularly water of different qualities. Throughout history, humans and animals alike have recognized the difference between various water sources and prefer those with a higher structure. Such a preference is visible with the Nazca (or Nasca) Lines, which date back around 100 B.C. to 650 A.D. The Nazca Lines are famous giant geoglyphs, easily etched into the surface of ground by moving away the top layer of stone, revealing the lighter color underneath. These lines maintain their integrity in the dry desert climate, and create giant geometric forms, parallel and crisscrossing lines, or animal and plant based symbols.

The longest line is nine miles long, and the shapes that are formed are only visible from the air. The lines were a contested topic for over 70 years, as historians and archaeologists argued about their purpose and function with all kinds of theories. It wasn't until intense investigation conducted by the Nazca Lines Project revealed an incredible discovery: the Nazca Lines were connected with subterranean springs and rivers, as well as above ground sources of water.

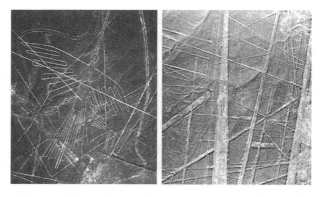

Fig. 14: Nazca Lines. Left: Aerial view of one of Nazca's giant geoglyphs. Right: Aerial view of part of the Nazca Lines complex.

As a desert based culture, water was the most central and important aspect of the Nazca culture. Also part of their culture were long processions, which involved walking great distances across the desert and along the Nazca Lines. These lines would direct the people to different sources and qualities of water, as well as mark subsurface water springs and channels. Their system of marking the sources, actions, and differences of water in their environment was precise: different geometric structures represented different types of water sources, whether underground aquifers and aqueducts, springs, or channels. Different structures and lines also notated the different zones of permeability in the ground, defining the areas of land capable of transmitting ground water as well as the location of water flow boundaries. For example, trapezoids lay over veins and distributary channels beneath the stony ground, while triangular shapes pointed to different sources of water. Some lines indicate where the water table would be high enough for digging wells or collecting water seepage. As a collective, the Nazca Lines essentially created a physical map on the surface of the ground for the drainage of subsurface water.[3]

There is virtually no rainfall in the Nazca desert, so this veneration of water comes as no surprise. And yet we mention the Nazca Lines within the context of structured water because of the strong indications that the Nazca people would walk miles across the desert to reach a specific water source – even if they were already located near one that was producing water, or if it meant passing others on the way. Water sources with higher mineral content and greater oxygen sources were sought out across great distances. The Nazca people knew the value of water, and they preferred structured sources, to the extent of marking gigantic symbols and walkways to mark their location. Because there is so little rainfall in the Nazca Valley, nearly all of the water sources from drainage paths noted by the Nazca people are the draining routes of melted ice from meteors, potentially creating a broad range in water quality. Some water

3. Mabee, S. and Proulx, D. The Correlation Between Geoglyphs and Subterranean Water Resources in the Rio Grande de Nazca Drainage. *Andean Archaeology II: Art, Landscape and Society.* New York: Kluwer Academic/Plenum Publishers. 2002.

sources do originate from the little rainfall Nazca Valley receives, but the site at Cerro Colorado, revered by the Nazca people and marked by a huge geoglyph, has a unique chemical signature that suggests it has some unknown source. With their great dependence, awareness, and sensitivities to water, the Nazca culture was knowledgeable of the difference in quality between waters of different structural levels. They operated the central theme of their water-based culture around recognizing these different sources of water, and making painstaking pilgrimages across the desert to access such quality and high structured sources.[4]

Much evidence from ancient cultures, such as those responsible for the construction of the Sphinx, the Giza Pyramids, or even the ancient pyramid structures off the coast of Japan and elsewhere across the globe, are lost to us today. However, there is still an abundance of information relating to more recent cultures and their guarded traditions, including descriptions of their relationship with water and their practices of 'water-preaching'. The Shinto religion of Japan is one such example. While most people living in Japan actually consider themselves 'non-religious', approximately 80% of the country also consider themselves *Shintoists*, following the way of life described in the Shinto tradition, making it Japan's traditional religion. The Shinto practice involves concepts of impurity and impure actions (i.e. sin or negative karma) that are cleansed from the individual with water rituals for purification. Only natural running water is used, in the forms of rivers, springs, and waterfalls, the latter being preferred. Prayers are recited multiple times to the water, both before the water cleansing and during, invoking the consciousness

4. Proulx, D. *The Nasca Lines Project*. University of Massachusetts. Web. 2001.

information of their prayers into the pattern of the water. Knowing how prayers and consciousness affect water, we see that Shinto water rituals are really based on the premise of structuring the water used during ceremony. In Japanese Buddhism, which is practiced alongside Shinto, as both are considered to be a way of life rather than religious systems and are not in contradiction to each other, a *tsukubai,* or small water basin, is provided in the front of the Buddhist temples for ritual purifications, or ablutions, prior to entering the temple or attending a tea ceremony.

Other water-based religions, cultures, and tribes also used water as the way of purification and spiritual cleanliness, as well as for divination. While the details of their belief systems and water-practices were not shared with outsiders and rarely survived antiquity, it is known that clan and tribe leaders or council members were often given the title 'High Water Priestess', which was a position passed down from mother to daughter (or sister), as is the case with the Water Priestesses of the Oru-Igbo tribe in Africa, or the Pegae Water Priestesses of Ancient Egypt. The High Water Priestess, which serves as both the spiritual leader and the clan leader, is a post held only by women, usually based on the belief that the divine ability to interpret divination and to influence the water is stronger in the female.

Water divination rituals were traditionally closely guarded, but likely include water scrying and steam divination, practices common among water-based religions. These rituals are highly based on structured water's responsiveness. Scrying rituals usually involve sacred water (highly structured) placed in specific bowls, typically made out of stone or crystal. Crystals and minerals are resonant with the frequencies and harmonic energies of Earth (being from Earth themselves), and thus will resonate (vibrate harmonically, or in sync) with the conscious meditation state of the individual performing the divination. Quartz-based bowls were most often used, the likely reason being these ancient groups recognized the energetic relationship and harmony of quartz crystal and water – their molecular structures are based on geometries that fit together perfectly, allowing for resonant information transfer. The one performing the divination, such as the Water Priestesses of Ancient Egypt, enters into a state of connection with the Water. She is then able to see symbols manifested out of the depths of the water, which may cloud or move in its actions with the diviner. These symbols, images, or events are then interpreted correctly by her divine ability. Steam divination involves, of course, the use of steam, which may reveal symbols or patterns in the clouds as it rises and as the fog or condensation drips onto crystal or mirrored surfaces involved in the ritual.

Here we see a strong connection with structured water and consciousness principles. In its active response to consciousness as a highly structured liquid crystal, the water adjusts its molecular structure to express certain information. The one performing the divination is in a state of coherent consciousness, their brainwave patterns and electrical firings rhythmically vibrating in synchronization, phase, and harmony, for coherent information processing. Entering into a state of connection with the water, they establish a resonant frequency exchange. Being in a highly resonant state already, composed primarily of highly structured water, it is possible for trained individuals and/or ones endowed with 'divine ability' to resonate harmonically with the highly structured water used for the ceremony. With harmonic resonance between the individual and the water comes high information transfer, thus the one performing the divination is able to gather information, in the form of symbols expressed in the water itself – through its structural expression – symbols that are able to be interpreted correctly by the high consciousness of the individual, which expresses itself with a level of coherency adequate enough to process the information gained from the interaction with the water, the result being a correct interpretation, answer, or foresight.

Another example of a water-based religious group is the Mandaeans, a sect of Gnostics that are still alive today. While the dates of their origins are uncertain, we do know that they migrated to Mesopotamia in the first century C.E. and are most certainly of pre-Arab and pre-Islamic origin, said to be the "remnants of the Jewish tribes who remained in Babylonia when other tribes left it for Jerusalem."[5] They are the indigenous Mandaic community of Iraq, with a pre-Iraq War population of 60-70,000 people, a population that has largely collapsed and relocated to nearby Iran, Syria, and Jordan. The Mandaeans themselves attest that they are direct descendants of Noah (and thus Adam), and revere John the Baptist as one of their greatest teachers. Their beliefs and practices are based on purity and purification, and the group originates from Gnostism, *manda* also meaning 'knowledge' or 'knowledge of life' much like the word *gnosis*. They were also commonly referred to by a slang term by outsiders in the Middle East, which translates literally to "the Baptizers". As their nickname and reverence for John the Baptist implies, the Mandaeans are strong Water-preachers, devoted to the practice of

5. Drower, E.S. *The Mandaeans of Iraq and Iran*. Leiden: Brill. 1962.

baptism as a way of spiritual purification for enlightenment.

> *They are a very simply people and they claim to posses a secret law of God...They wash day and night so as not to be condemned by God...*
> ~RICOLDO DA MONTECROCE, 1290 A.D.

An incredibly secretive group, the knowledge of ancient rites, rituals, certain sacred texts, and water practices are strictly reserved for those initiated as priests and priestesses of the Mandaeans. Priests and Priestesses of the community who have been fully initiated, who have attained access to the secret books and teachings, who observe strictly the rules of ritual purity, and who understand the secret doctrine, are called *Nasoreans, Nazarenes, Nazarean,* or *Nazorenes,* (used with a 'z' when emphasized). The word has its origins in the Hebrew word *nazir,* meaning 'consecrated' or 'separated', and is used in modern times to refer to monks.[6] The term *Nazorite* or *Nazarite* refers to one who voluntarily takes a vow described in the Old Testament Numbers 6:1, to follow specific rules of purity for a designated length of time, at the end of which was performed a ritual of initiation as a Nazarite Priest. Initiation involved the immersion of the individual in a *mikevah* or *mikvah,* a Jewish bath of purification and a baptism that involves immersing in a body of 'Living Waters', a repetitive phrase and theme we will examine in the next chapter. It is written that John the Baptist was a Nazarite from birth, making his vow of purity lifelong. Nazarites were considered to be holy men, especially favored and given grace by God, and "more pure than driven snow...more

6. Drower, E.S. *The Secret of Adam.* New York: Oxford University Press. 1960.

ruddy in body than rubies, their polishing was of sapphire..." (Old Testament Lamentations 4:7). It was believed they were honored and blessed by God for attaining purity and Priesthood by choice, rather than being forced into the role by birth (as was the case with the Tribe of Levi). A *Nazarite* is distinctly different from a *Nazorene*, as not all Nazarite Priests had attained high enough consciousness, purity, and understanding to access the sacred and secret teachings. Thus, the title of *Nasorean* or *Nazorene* was granted only to those who had reached this level. John the Baptist was most certainly considered a Nazarene, fully initiated to the secret teachings of the Nazarites.[7]

While the City of Nazareth appears from historical records to have gotten its name from the fact that many Nazarite Priests lived in the area, many residents of Nazareth were *not* Nazarites, and there is great debate on whether or not the city of Nazareth was even called such during Jesus's time. The City of Nazareth is not found in any book, map, chronicle, or military record of the time, with no epigraphic or archaeological evidence appearing until at least 60 or 70 CE. Thus, it was not a common or even accepted form of naming to refer to someone as being 'of Nazareth' (as in 'Jesus of Nazareth'), particularly when the Hebrew word *nazir* is specific in its association with being 'consecrated', 'devoted', 'separate', 'crowned', or 'of monk status'. Because of this, there are several Christian scholars who assert that Jesus was more likely called *'Jesus the Nazarene'* (also spelled Nazorean, Nazorene, Nazarene, or Nazarean) as it says in the Book of Matthew, not because he spent part of his life in the

7. Segelberg, Eric. *The Ordination of the Mandaean tarmida and its Relation to Jewish and Early Christian Ordination Rights.* Oxford International Conference on Patristic Studies: Studia Patristica, 10. 1970.

City of Nazareth, but rather as a reference to the status that Jesus held as one who knew, understood, and practiced the secret doctrine. The secret doctrine of the Mandaean Nazorenes is heavily rooted in structured Water rituals and is the hidden knowledge of spiritual purity, enlightenment, and the attainment of everlasting life or ascension – where one attains such a high level of consciousness that they are no longer imprisoned in the material body and the material self, finally able to 'ascend' or rise to a higher dimensional existence, i.e. Heaven or Nirvana. As these are all actions and abilities attributed to Jesus Christ, it seems plausible that the title *Jesus the Nazarene* really was in reference to the spiritual purity, enlightenment, everlasting life, and ascension abilities that Jesus possessed, making him a true *Nazarene,* or *Nazorene*, spelled with a 'z' to display the emphatic use of the term.

The baptism practices and water rituals of the Mandaeans were not uncommon among other Gnostic groups or even the Hebrews, who also held great reverence for Water. These groups engaged in water baptisms on a regular basis, as virtually every sacred ceremony or ritual that was conducted involved ritual cleansing practices before it was performed. In ancient Hebrew Temple times, for example, the priests as well as each pilgrim who wished entry into the Holy Temple built by King Solomon had to first immerse themselves in a *mikvah,* or body of living waters. On the Hebrew holy day of Yom Kippur, the high priest was allowed entrance into the Holy of Holies, the innermost chamber of the temple and the room where the sacred Ark of the Covenant was kept, a place that no other mortal could enter. In order to enter the sacred space of the temple, he was required to perform a number of preparation services or rituals, each of which was preceded by immersion in the *mikvah* bath of living waters.

The healing power of immersion in living water or of other water rituals has offered a literal and spiritual gateway to purity ever since the creation of humankind. It is the most common medium of purification, is considered to have an intrinsic purity and the capacity to absorb both physical and energetic pollution and carry it away. The anti-bacterial and anti-pollution properties are the literal and physical applications of Water's cleansing and purification properties, and are reflective of its abilities to cleanse the energetic, conscious, spiritual, and soulful realm as taught by water-based religions and teachers throughout antiquity.

CHAPTER 20

# LIVING WATERS, WATERS OF LIFE:

## WHAT WATER BASED RELIGIONS REALLY TEACH

*The Upholder of the Cycles which supports the whole of Life, is water. In every drop of water dwells the Godhead, whom we all serve; there also dwells Life, the Soul of the First substance – Water – whose boundaries and banks are the capillaries that guide it and in which it circulates.*
~VIKTOR SCHAUBERGER

While it is clear that water rituals, baptisms, and sin and spiritual cleansing were an integral part of multiple religious traditions, in order to understand the meaning behind these practices as deeper than mere symbolism and grasp how richly connected to the real science and physics of our reality they are, we need to have a better understanding of what these various traditions reveal about their knowledge of water's amazing abilities and functions, and what their teachings reveal about the relationship between God, consciousness, spirituality, everlasting life, and Water. To do this, we must reach back into the ancient texts and teachings that have survived history and re-read them within the context of this discussion, where we find the expressions of this knowledge within their texts and teachings, beginning with virtually every tradition connecting Water with the beginning of Life.

*We have created every living thing from water.*
~QUR'AN: SURA 21 THE PROPHETS, AYAT 30

*...Let the waters bring forth abundantly the moving creature that hath life...*
BIBLE, OLD TESTAMENT: GENESIS 1:20

*The whole Universe is made up of water.*
*All beings are made up of water.*
*The vital airs, are the effects of water;*
*cows are also the effect of water,*
*food comes from water, all the kingdoms, cosmos,*
*Vedic metres, all are made of water;*
*water is truth and all the deities are water,*
*all the worlds are made up of water.*
~VEDIC TEXT, MAHANARAYANA UPANISHAD 4.29

The above scriptures are examples from the three largest world religions, Islam, Hindu, and Christianity. The central texts of Hinduism, called *Vedic texts*, are actually comprised of a large number of writings originating from ancient India which combined creates several volumes worth of work. *Veda* is the Sanskrit word for *knowledge,* and this compilation of texts can be of particular interest for their wide range of information. Their inherent knowledge and understandings of science, biology, physics, and mathematics is unparalleled in the ancient world, and the Vedic texts reveal clear understandings of the Earth's water cycles, with accurate detailed explanations of the processes of evaporation, condensation, rain, and cloud formation thousands of years before they were recognized by classes and disciplines of science. In the above Vedic scripture, we see that the wisdom keepers and sages of their times also knew that we were all made of water, something modern science has only recently realized, now recognizing that 99% of our molecules are, in fact, water. Yet centuries ago we were known without question to have come from water. The Vedic texts, such as the Upanishad excerpt above, took this further in the statement that *the whole universe is made up of water...* This type of statement carries much more importance when we look at what type of information can be or is stored in water's molecular structure, and how this occurs. We know the whole Universe is *not* made up of water; there are of course other elements abundant in space, as well as 'space' itself and the mysterious 'dark matter' and 'dark energy', which account for most of our Universe. But we also know that water is crystallographic and *highly changeable,* that it has a dynamic relationship with consciousness, and that it acts, in a sense, as a 'record keeper' – encoding and storing information into its structural arrangement. Today, the most advanced sciences discuss theories on the crystallographic nature of the Universe, a topic we have already covered. These theories emphasize the crystallographic nature to the background of our physical Universe, and the connection between consciousness, energy, and the Universe, wherein our Universe (and everything in it) is viewed as different expressions of *consciousness,* and thus has a dynamic relationship with *our* consciousness (giving rise to such principles as the Law of Attraction, wherein our consciousness has a direct effect on our manifested reality). Because our Universe also appears to function on principles of *holography,* wherein each small piece contains all the information of the whole, we see in this way that the crystallographic patterns of our Universe also act, in a sense, as a 'record keeper'. With these facts in mind, the Vedic teaching that *"the whole Universe is water..."* may actually be pointing to the greater truth about the flexible and responsive nature of our crystallographic Universe.

The script continues, *"Water is truth..."* Water, in its intelligent processing of all forms of information, does not lie and cannot be tricked. If someone speaks the word 'Love' but thinks the word 'Hate', the water is not fooled; it will reflect the consciousness of the thought, and within the context of the spoken lie. These will be expressed as complex geometric forms, carrying the layers of information behind any particular consciousness – the intention, the motivation, the history of cause and effect that created the situation – *all* this information is decoded and expressed in the Water's multi-dimensional and fractal crystallographic patterns. Water, most certainly, reflects truth.

*"...and all the deities are water..."* Deities can generally be thought of as archetypes, or embodiments of certain characteristics, who have great and expanded abilities. They can represent specific virtues or traits, which express a powerful and complex energetic pattern. Archetypes, virtues, great and expanded abilities, and certain characteristics are reflective of specific patterns. Certain geometric structures allow energy to move in a certain way, giving rise to different physical manifestations, and allowing for different interactions

with the environment. These specific patterns are also emblematic of a respective level, or type, of consciousness – that is to say, certain geometric patterns will express different aspects of consciousness or human/deity natures, which gives rise to the differences in personalities and abilities associated with these various characters. We can see this concept readily within the Tibetan Buddhist tradition, where the Dalai Lama (the title given to their appointed leader) is viewed as a reincarnation of a specific entity, the Bodhisattva (or enlightened being) of Compassion, thus his personality, abilities, and messages center around a theme of compassion. There are also, however, the Bodhisattva's of Wisdom, of Infinite Happiness, of Meditation, of Protection, of Abundance, etc. In this manner, we can see that the virtues associated with a specific 'Bodhisattva' archetype are emblematic of an overriding *pattern,* and that the Dalai Lama as the reincarnate Bodhisattva of Compassion has this overriding pattern within his water system and/or consciousness, giving rise to the certain manifestations of personality and character. The Dalai Lama cares greatly about compassion and recognizes its importance as a pattern of consciousness, and thus preaches this message to the world. In this perspective, we recognize that the Dalai Lama carries within his individual pattern arrangement a specific geometric pattern that is connected with compassion. Also in this way, we can understand the deeper message behind the Vedic text *"all the deities are water..."* for truly the respective patterns of all deities or archetypes can be found in water, and the expanded abilities of all deities arise from a coherent crystallographic structure.

This Vedic scripture is certainly not the only one to make such dramatic statements about water, or to imply what type of information can be or is stored in its molecular structure. Much like the Upanishad's implication that all the deities are water, we find that water is recognized as a vessel of God, Spirit, Christ, or Prana in virtually every ancient tradition – Prana being the Sanskrit term for a vital life force, often synonymous with the Chinese concept of Qi or Chi and and the Japanese concept of Ki, as in 'Reiki'. In the same way that compassion can be interpreted as a specific geometric structure, so too can the pattern of God, by any name, and the virtues of Jesus Christ, Buddha, or Krishna be viewed as specific geometric structure.

This is how we understand that water can carry the Spirit of God – wherein it has the ability to express the God consciousness, or Christ consciousness, in a non-entropic structure that is perfect in its geometric complexity and arrangement, expressing the total and complete coherence that elevate consciousness to a transcendent level of being. Waters that hold Prana, Chi, or the Spirit of God are also called *Living Waters* or *Waters of Life*. The references to such *Living Water* are innumerable within the ancient spiritual literature, appearing in a variety of traditions across the world.

*For My people have forsaken Me, [God] the fountain of living waters...*
~BIBLE, OLD TESTAMENT: JEREMIAH 2:13

*Water, when drunk, becomes divided into three parts. What is its grossest ingredient, that becomes urine, what is the middling ingredient, that becomes blood, and what is the subtlest ingredient, that becomes Prana...Hence dear boy, mind is made up of food, Prana is made up of water, and speech is made of fire. 'Explain it further to me, revered sir'. 'Be it so,*

*dear boy,' said the father...Dear boy, of the water that is drunk
that which is the subtlest part rises upwards and that becomes
Prana.*
~THE CHANDOGYA UPANISHAD: VI,V-2 – VI,VI-3

*And he shewed me a pure river of water of life, clear as
crystal, proceeding out of the throne of God and of the Lamb.*
~BIBLE, NEW TESTAMENT: REVELATION 22:1

*I have reached the inner vision and through Thy Spirit in
me I have heard Thy wondrous secret, through Thy mystic
insight Thou hast caused a spring of knowledge to well up
within me, a fountain of power, pouring forth living waters, a
flood of love and of all embracing wisdom, like the splendour of
eternal light.*
~BOOK OF HYMNS, DEAD SEA SCROLLS

*In the midst of the Waters is moving the Lord, surveying
men's truth and men's lies.*
~RIG VEDA VII, 49

Above we see that in Judeo-Christian literature, God
calls Himself the *"fountain of living waters,"* and that the
last chapter of the New Testament describes a *"pure river
of water of life, proceeding out of the throne of God..."* This
is the holiest of holy Water, structured with the perfect
spirit of God – perfect geometries which experience no
entropy or decay, and are thus the Waters of Life. It is a
common theme, also expressed in the following passages
of Christian scripture:

*But whosoever drinketh of the water that I shall give him
shall be in him a well of water springing up into everlasting
life.*

~BIBLE, NEW TESTAMENT: JOHN 4:14

*He that believeth on me, as the scripture hath said, out of his belly shall flow rivers of living water.*
~BIBLE, NEW TESTAMENT: JOHN 7:38

Here we see a common description in Christianity of the recognition of *living waters* and the connection between *believing and drinking the water of Christ, rivers of living water in the belly of a man,* and *water causing everlasting life.* When we consider that the belly, the seat of the solar plexus chakra and a major energetic center, is connected here to flowing rivers of living water, we are able to view the scripture from a bio-energetic standpoint. When we understand that *meridians* are synonymous with *rivers of energy in the body,* the scripture has a deeper meaning on a physical and bio-energetic level than the simple metaphor that is commonly relayed in popular Christianity. Learning from the Upanishads, we see that Prana, the vital life force, is made of water. In this context, the scripture now reads that from the solar plexus Prana will distribute throughout the body, bringing *rivers of living waters* throughout the meridian system, and delivering the vital force of Life to the body. When this water, as a vessel of God, carries the *perfect structure* of Christ and God, it becomes a spring of *everlasting life,* bringing constant, renewed waters through the *well springing up* and the *flowing rivers.* Relating this knowledge to our scientific grasp of cellular life, we suddenly see that discussions of water as part of the key to everlasting life are perhaps not so metaphorical. Recall again Dr. Carrel's statement:

*The cell is immortal. It is merely the fluid in which*

*it floats that degenerates. Renew this fluid at regular intervals, give the cells what they require for nutrition, and as far as we know, the pulsation of life can go on forever.*
~DR. ALEXIS CARREL
NOBEL PRIZE, PHYSIOLOGY OR MEDICINE

When we acknowledge that the structure of water is the Essence of all Life, that the integrity and life-span of the DNA is *dependent* on the structure of its surrounding water, and that renewing the cellular fluids at regular intervals *with the geometrically complex structured water is all it requires to be continually sustained,* all lessons taught to us by science, we can understand how complexly structured water in our bodies – water that does not become de-structured and de-natured by entropic forces in our environment, or water that has *overcome* these entropic forces in our environment – *could indeed be a well-spring of everlasting life.* Here, Christian literature is expressing to us that the key to everlasting life, the way to renew the waters in the body, the subtle-energy of Prana, and the cellular fluid at regular intervals, is to have encoded into the structure of the bio-water the complex geometric patterns created by Christ, i.e. *the complex geometric pattern of the embodiment of God consciousness in Man.*

*As the smallest drop of water detached from the ocean contains all the qualities of the ocean, so man, detached in consciousness from the Infinite, contains within him its likeness; and as the drop of water must, by the law of its nature, ultimately find its way back to the ocean and lose itself in its silent depths, so must man, by the unfailing law of his nature, at last return to his source, and lose himself in the great ocean of the Infinite.*
~JAMES ALLEN, AUTHOR, PHILOSOPHER

CHAPTER 21

# LESSONS IN THE WATER PRAYERS

---

As water is highly responsive to consciousness, it is no wonder that cultures have been blessing their water in the name of their God, and thus structuring it and changing its properties, since antiquity. It is perhaps one of the oldest traditions among the various religions of the world.

*Ceaselessly they flow from the depths, pure, never sleeping,*
*the Ocean their sponsor,*
*Following the channels ordained by the Thunderer.*
*Now may these great divine Waters quicken me!*
*Waters may pour from heaven*
*or run along channels dug out by men;*
*Or flow clear and pure having the Ocean as their goal.*
*Now may these great divine Waters quicken me!*
*In the midst of the Waters is moving the Lord,*
*surveying men's truth and men's lies.*
*How sweet are the Waters, crystal clear and cleansing!*
*Now may these great divine Waters quicken me!*
*...Into whom the Universal Lord has entered,*
*Now may these great divine Waters quicken me!*
~RIG VEDA, VII 49

The Vedic and Hindu prayer above eloquently demonstrates the culture's knowledge of and reverence for Water. It speaks of the Lord being in the water, *surveying men's truth and men's lies*. In its connection and reflection of consciousness, this is another description of the abilities of structured water, to survey (and record) "men's truth and men's lies". As we discussed earlier, Water has the ability through its incredible responsiveness and resonant information transfer to decode and express infinite information. The Vedic scripture teaches that the Lord is *in* the midst of the Waters, conducting the force of its structure as the expression of His movement. Here we also see Water described as *Into whom the Universal Lord has entered*. Once again we see the expression of the presence of God entering Water, the physics of which is displayed in the complex structure of holy waters.

The following is another Vedic prayer to Water:

*O Waters, source of happiness, pray give us vigor*
*so that we may contemplate the great delight.*
*You like loving mothers are who long to give children dear.*
*Give us of your propitious sap. On your behalf we desire, O*
*Waters,*
*To assist the one to whose house you send us –*
*you, of our life and being the source,*
*These Waters be to us for drink; divine are they for aid and*
*joy.*
*May they impart to us health and strength!*
*You Waters who rule over precious things and have*
*supreme control of men, we beg you, give us healing balm.*
*Within the Waters, Soma has told me,*

> *Remedies exist of every sort and Agni who brings blessing to*
> *all.*
> *O Waters, stored with healing balm*
> *through which my body safe will be,*
> *Come that I long may see the sun.*
> *Whatever sin is found in me, whatever wrong I may have*
> *done,*
> *If I have lied or falsely sworn, Waters, remove it far from*
> *me.*
> *Now I have come to seek the Waters.*
> ~RIG VEDA X, 9

This prayer, when read carefully, expresses much in its meaning. We find that the Vedas believed Water to have *supreme control of men*, and to be able to provide *healing balm*. It further states that *Within the Waters...Remedies exist of every sort, and Agni who brings blessing to all.* "Agni" is Sanskrit for "fire" or "fire of God", thus the scripture is telling us that *both* remedies of *every* sort *and* the spirit or fire of God exists within the waters. *O Waters, stored with healing balm,* refers to the structure literally stored within the water, and in effect is similar to homeopathy, in that the structure of the water certainly *can* heal.

The closing of this prayer is perhaps the most compelling part. *Whatever sin is found in me, whatever wrong I may have done, If I have lied or falsely sworn, Waters, remove it far from me.* Viewing this scripture through they eyes of structured bio-water consciousness, we see that the Vedic sages are telling us that *Water can remove sin.* The prayer says that *whatever* wrong one has done, water has the ability to remove it. This implies a necessary *re-coding* of the water's structure within the body, which would remove or undo the de-structured effect of what one would term as sin. *Whatever* sin may be found, be it any form of wrongdoing or lying, can be removed, re-coded, and re-structured back to higher form through the power of structured water. Through the language of the prayer, we see that the Vedics are invoking a great consciousness into their water, with acknowledgement and gratitude for Water as the source of happiness, the carrier of every remedy, and a vessel for Agni and the fire of God. *It is this high structure created through the consciousness of their prayer that allows for the blessed water to remove their sin.*

This is also the role that a priest, minister, or spiritual being plays when he or she blesses water in preparation for baptism, a cleansing ritual not limited to Christianity but rather widespread as practices of immersion across virtually *every* culture. The effect of the prayer, intention, and the blessing of the water is the creation of a highly structured pattern, which has encoded the high consciousness of the prayer. Immersions, baptisms, and water purification rituals are performed to provide a 'cleansing of sin' or purification for righteousness, and to a lesser degree this is also the function of holy water used in churches and various uses of sacred waters in a variety of traditions.

*Then I will sprinkle clean water upon you, and ye shall be clean from all your filthiness, and from all your idols, will I cleanse you.*
~BIBLE, OLD TESTAMENT: EZEKIEL 36:25

*And now, why are you waiting? Arise and be baptized, and wash away your sins, calling on the name of the Lord.*
~BIBLE, NEW TESTAMENT: ACTS 22:16

*...but according to His mercy He saved us, through the*

*washing of regeneration and renewing of the Holy Spirit.*
~BIBLE, NEW TESTAMENT: TITUS 3:5

*Let us draw near with a true heart in full assurance of faith,*
*having our hearts sprinkled from an evil conscience*
*and our bodies washed with pure water.*
~BIBLE, NEW TESTAMENT: HEBREWS 10:22

The idea of water removing sin or cleansing karma is rather pervasive throughout human antiquity, and Christianity and Hinduism are, of course, only two examples of the many religions and cultures that use water in this way. It is a practice that today is rarely understood and often viewed as metaphor and symbolism of an ancient rite, ritual, or tradition, and rather than the basis for the effectiveness of the ritual itself. From a structured water perspective, this concept takes on much deeper physical and spiritual meanings.

Many people have undertaken the topic of defining sin and karma, and entire books have been written on the topic. For the sake of this conversation, I will give a brief definition that we may hopefully understand in order to continue with our discussion on water. Karma is often considered the result of action, both the positive and negative forces of cause and effect, which operate in the subtle energy laws of magnetism and attraction – wherein doing a 'bad deed' will eventually come back to you as something negative that manifests in your life, while doing a 'good deed' will eventually come back to you as manifesting something positive in your life. When discussed in the same context with sin, karma is often meant to relate to the negative aspect of cause and effect, the negativity that is attached to sin, or the sort of 'accumulated sin' one can experience as the karma they have 'built up'. Sin is often considered something we have done or thought that goes 'against God', or as some would say 'against Good' – essentially, it is something we judge ourselves negatively for, whether consciously or subconsciously, as not being the highest form of action we could have taken.

Consider the effects that our experiences, thoughts, actions, and our judgments of those experiences, thoughts, and actions, have on the structure of our water. Sin and Karma, both positive karma and negative karma, are stored as patterns within our water. Perhaps this is the reason for the long-held belief that we are born with the sins of our parents, or are born with karma from parents or previous lives – because of the patterns inherent in the structure of our water at birth. It is most certainly the reason that sin and karma are so often associated with the experience of disease and death – the de-structuring nature that negativity, as in negative thought patterns and consciousness, have on our water is what brings about physical disease, aging, and death. Consider the following passages that illustrate this point: Biblical scriptures state that Christ was *"manifested to take away our sins"* (1 John 3:5), and that sin is the power of death, *"The wages of sin is death"* (Rom. 6:23), and thus through taking away sins, in which lies the power of death, Christ came to destroy the power of death, *"... as the children are partakers of flesh and blood, he also likewise took part of the same; that through death he might destroy him that had the power of death..."* (Hebrews 2:14-15).

It is in this way that the Christ of Christianity came to fight death, abolish sin, and absolve Karma, by displaying the type of consciousness, faith, and knowledge necessary for the highest structure of waters, thus bringing everlasting life. Within this tradition, faith in Christ and God, and the absolute knowledge of forgiveness and perfection, allows one to release the negative energy stored in the structure of water, releasing and taking away sins, which alleviates the fear of death and any judgment. The patterns of water formed by the energy of a figure such as Christ are of the highest geometric complexity and integrity, supporting life, wellness, and consciousness. The term 'Christ Consciousness' or 'Krishna Consciousness' refers to a purified state of consciousness wherein one has incorporated the Spirit of Christ (or in the Spirit of Krishna, in its respective tradition) into their being, their spirit of consciousness having evolved to such a high degree that they are now beginning to emulate the Spirit of Christ or Krishna and the purity of consciousness within themselves, a reflection of the integration of the Christ energy and patterns within their own energetic and water structures.

> *For the Master, Jesus, even the Christ, is the pattern for every man in the Earth, whether he be Gentile or Jew, Parthenian or Greek. For all have the pattern, whether they call on that name or not; but there is no other name given under heaven whereby men may be saved from themselves.*
> ~EDGAR CAYCE, 3528-1

What Cayce echoes here is the sentiment that Christ represents a *pattern* for man to follow, and as we know in the world of geometric structures, it is all about the *patterns.* The words of Jesus, *"Verily, verily, I say unto you, He that believeth on me, the works that I do shall he do also; and greater works than these he will do..."* (John 14:12) represents as a whole the entire concept held within Christianity of

Jesus as a pattern for man. It holds massive implications, particularly when viewed through the context of structured water principles. The 'works' the verse is referring to include the witnessed 'miracles', i.e. the changing water into wine, the feeding of the 5,000, the raising of the dead, and multiple healings of the sick, diseased, and maimed.

*Therefore if any man be in Christ, he is a new creature: old things are passed away; behold, all things are become new.*
~BIBLE, NEW TESTAMENT: 2 CORINTHIANS 5:17

When we contend that the ability to cause massive changes in the structural system is what allows for the changing of water into wine, the ability for five loaves of bread to be continually divided to feed a mass group of people, immediate and 'miraculous' healings of disease and injury, and yes, even the raising of the dead or the reinvigorating of the flow and force of Life within the bio-water and energetic system, we realize that the miracles performed were in fact operating on structural principles. Christ, in attaining the highest structure attainable within the bio-waters, was able to affect, move, and direct energy in multiple ways. In understanding the physics of highly structured bio-waters, we recognize that upon attaining this level of structure within ourselves, we, too, would be able to move and manipulate subtle energy and structural information, the application of which would result in the 'miraculous' works. In achieving this highly structured, non-entropic pattern in our bio-waters, we would be free of death and disease, achieving freedom from the 'wages of sin' and defeating death in a similar manner to that described of the Christ.

Ancient knowledge and the science of structured water

show us the importance and effect of consciousness and energy, and a physical manifestation of the evolution of our consciousness through the change of structure in our bio-waters. Understanding that we are our water, we can begin to grasp the importance of what is stored within its structure. We can begin to see how our accumulated thoughts, actions, experiences, and perception and judgments – both judgments of others and of ourselves – are stored within the structure of our water and affect our physical experience of both life and death. We begin to understand that our water is not just our sea of consciousness and memory, *but also where our karma is stored*, playing out through our lives in the expression of particular patterns and structures, affecting our emotional, spiritual, and physical body and participating in the Magnetic Law of Attraction in the Universe, manifesting and drawing to the individual the experiences and perceptions which resonate with its form and programming.

Aging, death, and disease are a result of the de-structuring of our bio-waters, de-structuring that occurs because of exposure to pollution, toxins, and negative emotions or consciousness. Thus, re-structuring the water in our body is our only real means of combating the physical and energetic pollution in our environment, whether from our air, food, water, or electromagnetic pollution such as those generated by cell phones and computers, as well as our best means of combating the effects of negative thought patterns and judgments, clearing karma and releasing ourselves from the judgment of sins in order to evolve and advance our consciousness to a higher state of being, a higher state of consciousness, and a higher state of mental, emotional, energetic, and physical functioning. All of this means a greater connection to Spirit, and the ability to more greatly interact with the Laws of Positive Attraction, to see our intentions manifest in our experience. *Our path to greater consciousness, expanded awareness, deeper understandings, and longevity in prosperous health resides in the Structure of our Water – because our consciousness exists in and through our Water.*

This is really what it's all about. The connection of mankind to God or Spirit, and our soulful longing and desire to pursue questions of the spirit, comes from an ancient inner driving force that guides us towards these connections, based on an inner knowing that *this* is the ultimate fulfillment of experience. This inner driving force causes us to seek higher and higher levels of consciousness, which in turn breeds a greater sense of spirituality, awareness, and abilities, a greater knowingness of our connection to God, each other, and our world, and a sense past the illusion of duality and separation that defines our plane of physical reality. Consciousness, awareness, abilities, and knowledge – these are the ultimate attainment for the soul and spirit, and they are all a by-product of our water and intimately connected in a feedback system. We all want higher levels of consciousness so we can participate in the Law of Attraction positively, so we can escape our destructive habits or our inability to incorporate positive habits as much as we would like, so we can experience an enriched and full existence. In Life we are all searching for *more,* in our hearts, in our spirits, and in our experiences, and it comes only through the attainment of higher levels of consciousness – which is brought about through the structure of our Water. Because our Consciousness, and our Spirit, are held within our Water system.

# CHAPTER 22

# STRUCTURED WATER SCIENCE: REALIZING THE DREAM

---

The research and development in the field of structured liquid crystalline water and the structure of bio-waters and cellular fluids is phenomenal, and accumulating everyday. The support is overwhelming, despite the expected mainstream Western medicine and science dragging their feet. The implications are astounding, and are much too vast to possibly incorporate into one piece of work. It can, should, and eventually will revolutionize and transform healthcare and medicine, aging and life expectancy, disease treatment and prevention – including that of mental illness and genetic defects – psychology and psychiatry, healing sciences, agriculture, ecology, food production and preservation, water treatment and distribution, sanitation, education and development, relationships and human behavior, subtle energy sciences, homeopathy, consciousness studies, philosophy and theology, astrophysics, quantum physics and general physics, atomic and nuclear sciences, energy sources, unified field theories, progressive advancements in technologies, and quite literally improve *everyone's* quality of life. Never before has the understanding of a single substance and how it operates evaded scientists for so long. Never before has the revelation of what that single substance actually is, and the methods by which it does what it does, carried such enormous and incalculable implications that can affect virtually *every* aspect of our lives and every field of study. Never before has this single substance – the most abundant substance on Earth – been fully realized for its potentials. The effects are system-wide; Laws of Physics will be broken and left behind, as we enter a new world of discovery and achievement. We are at the cusp of a new era, the dawning of what will be the most groundbreaking innovations and developments ever before experienced, as paradigms are broken and we enter the greatest advent of the future – the age of structured water.

> *The revelation of the secret of water will put an end to all manner of speculation or expediency and their excrescences, to which belong war, hatred, impatience and discord of every kind. The thorough study of water therefore signifies the end of monopolies, the end of all domination in the truest sense of the word and the start of a socialism arising from the development of individualism in its most perfect form.*
>
> ~VIKTOR SCHAUBERGER, 1939

Perhaps this is the true meaning behind the foretelling of the great sages when they described the Age of Aquarius, which corresponds with other cultural traditions of the Golden Age, or the coming of the Kingdom on Earth. An 'Age' here simply refers to a period of time, as in the Bronze Age, the Stone Age, the Age of Enlightenment, etc. While the phrase 'Age of Aquarius' is practically laughable after the overplayed late 1960's rock song, it does refer to an actual zodiac and astrological age.

The Golden Age of the Maya is a separately calculated epoch that is generally interpreted as correlating with the transition to the Age of Aquarius, as do the general interpretations regarding the Biblical End of Days and the rule of Christ on Earth. Different astrological ages, such as the Age of Aquarius, exist as a result of precession of the equinoxes, in which the position of the sun as it rises above the celestial equator at the time of the spring equinox is marked by the zodiacal constellation over which it rises. The zodiacal constellation in place at the celestial equator at the time of the vernal equinox (spring equinox) changes every 2,150 years or so as the Earth travels through space. Thus, the 'age' is generally thought of as lasting approximately 2,150 years and defined by the zodiacal constellation to which it is associated. Astrologers associated specific 'ages' with expressions of development and cultural tendencies, and have widely varying interpretations on what each 'age' expresses or might bring, as well as widely varying calculations on when each age actually begins or ends – as constellations do not necessarily have well-defined 'borders' and in fact occasionally overlap, leading to speculation on when an actual transition from one age to the next has occurred. The general consensus is that transitions from one age to the next are a gradual process, and that the transition to the Age of Aquarius happens somewhere around the 20th century.

While the name may be just a coincidence and the Age of Aquarius just a fanciful idea held by a variety of cultures, the science of structured water and structured bio-water is as real and as viable as it gets. The answer to accomplishing our most sought after achievements – easy, accurate, and successful medical treatment and disease prevention, increased longevity, health, and quality of our experience of life, free energy and sustainable, reliable, renewable energy sources and clean water – lies in the most pervasive substance in the Universe. When the great sages said, 'the answer is right in front of you,' or 'the answer lies within you,' they were absolutely right.

Everyone dreams of a world where there is freedom from suffering, conflict, fear, disease, death, desperation, and demand. At one point in our lives, we all inherently dreamed of the same thing, a sentiment reflected in so many children across the world whose hope and innocence are still largely intact. We dreamed that all the people of the world would exist in peace, and not want for food and water nor live outside of perfect health and wellness. We dreamed that every disease could be cured, every injury healed, and every polluted ecosystem cleansed. These dreams are the voices of humanity's powerful collective consciousness and experience. When the full potentials of structured water and structured bio-waters are realized, so too will the dreams of humanity, and Life will become an entirely different experience.

When people begin to drive and demand change and innovation in the world relating to structured water and structured bio-water applications, then expansion and development will happen at an exponential rate. It will need to be the people who motivate such a movement, for it will not be motivated, at least not initially, by the pocketbooks of profit-driven groups like big pharma, big oil, and big business. Still, even these industries recognize that the race is on, and that the developments in the areas of science using structured water applications and therapies are inevitably showing themselves on the horizon of accomplishment, waiting for our achievement of them so that they may rise like the sun and shine their light on the world. When this happens, and we begin to fully apply the incredible potentials of structured water science, humanity will see and experience our reality in an entirely new way, and all of mankind will enter in a new day.

# PART V

# INSTRUCTIONS FROM NATURE

Through our brief exploration into the science and spirituality of water, we see the incredible importance of the structure of water, particularly our body's water. It is imperative in our physical processes – the structure of our bio-water determines the conductivity and the electromagnetic field interactions of our cells and DNA, it is vitally important in virtually *every* process in the body, and the *de-structuring* of our bio-water is intimately related to aging, disease, and death. The structure of our water determines the level of functioning in our brain and thought processes (our level of coherence), our ability to store, retrieve, and relate memories and experiences, and our capacity to recognize, interpret, and operate pattern recognition in our lives on various levels. Deeper yet, the structure of our water is directly related to the expansion of our consciousness, our level of awareness, the health of our spirituality, and, ultimately, our connection to God and our ability to manifest in our environment through the laws of attraction.

Science has long known this fundamental aspect of our physical health, and our ancestors throughout antiquity have known even longer still the great connection between water, energy, consciousness, and ultimately God or Source. Yet in today's advanced age, with *countless* pharmaceutical drugs and interventions, and a growing community of alternative, natural, and holistic therapies, there have been very few methods that are specifically targeted at re-structuring the body's water. Until 2009, in fact, there were none. And yet every natural method of healing, including meditation, light, magnetic, sound, or other energy therapies, have unknowingly operated to change the structure of the water in the body and have thus had wide beneficial effects. Light therapies have been used for centuries and have well-established effects on cellular function and bioactivity, hence the widespread adoption of light therapy lamps in neo-natal units to treat jaundice. Sound therapy, magnetic treatments, electromagnetic frequency therapies, consciousness treatments – including practices like neuro-linguistic programming, mantras, and positive thinking – internal or ingested remedies, and any form of subtle energy treatment, is affecting and changing the patterns, structure, and information stored in the water of the body. If such a therapy is successful, it means the individual has been able to fully integrate more complex forms of crystallographic patterns into the water of the body and improve the state of health. This improvement may even be temporary, as continuous exposure to negative internal and external environments and pollution continues to affect the structure of the water, and such exposure likely caused the de-structuring of the bio-waters to begin with (which in turn caused the physical symptoms and expression of dis-ease). The natural treatment practice of Homeopathy is most closely linked to structured water therapies, as it operates on principles of structuring water with the energetic structural pattern or signature of the remedy, and the structured water thus becomes the medicine. However, homeopathy is not targeting the waters of the body or specifically dealing with its geometric complexity, it is associating properties of the remedy's structural signatures with particular symptoms of disease. The field of intentionally structuring the water in the cellular systems has been relatively non-existent, with the exception of very few drinking water systems or the old adage of positive thinking and intention.

Unfortunately in today's polluted environments and stressful lifestyles, positive thinking and/or the ingestion of water that has been structured using intention or artificial means are insufficient to dramatically affect the structure of the water in the body. Intentionally structured water is still subjected to and affected by our ongoing mental and emotional states, as well as subject to rapid influence by the electromagnetic frequencies and radiations in an environment – not to mention the effect of plastics and the loss of integrity during transportation. However, now that there has been a significant breakthrough in development, more people have begun to explore the importance of this approach to health and a newly opened field is rapidly expanding. This expansion is occurring at an astounding rate as the anomalous behavior of water and its critical effect on cellular structures becomes more widely recognized and accepted.

The changing and responsive nature of the structure of water is becoming nearly impossible to ignore within the scientific community, at least not without displaying a large amount of ignorance. We have already seen some examples of how magnetism and different electromagnetic frequencies affect the structure of water, how we are able to observe newly acquired properties and effects like altering seed germination rates and plant growth, anti-bacterial properties, enzyme function, and DNA transference. And while these are all recognized ways of affecting the structure of water *outside* of the body, they provide insight into the ways to affect the structure *inside* the body as well. For this discussion, we will be highlighting the primary natural methods of re-structuring and intentionally excluding un-natural processes, which typically use electrocution and electric ionization methods. Most water treatment systems and structured water marketers use these methods, and they are incredibly de-structuring, rather than re-structuring, as their marketers would have you believe. Obviously electro-shock therapy was not an effective way of re-structuring the bio-waters, or it would have been a more successful therapy system. Similarly, electro-shocking water breaks apart its bonds and molecular structures without providing information necessary to reform those structures in highly complex repeating geometries, freeing hydrogen ions and resulting in an increased pH reading while destroying the structural integrity.

CHAPTER 23

# LIGHT

---

*I am remembering Water that glows in the dawn.*
~UNKNOWN

In 2005 a collaborative group of individuals from
various University Medical Centers and NASA
conducted a study to research the effects of various colors
on the properties of water. Bottles of distilled water were
wrapped in cellophane of either violet, indigo, blue,
green, yellow, orange, or red – the primary colors of the
visible spectrum and the associated colors of each of the
seven chakras in Ayurvedic tradition – and exposed to
sunlight for forty days, after which they were evaluated
for changes in properties. Different color-treated water
exhibited different effects on the "altered elemental
composition" of the water, or its structural changes,
changes in electrical conductance, osmolarity (solute
concentration) and salt-solubility, differences in bio-
modulatory effects (reactive adjustments in the
biochemical or cellular status), and accelerated and
increased root elongation in seed germination. Some of
the results were quite astonishing, leading to the

development of theories that solar energy is stored in the water as kinetic energy – similar to our understanding of the storage of pattern information that can allow for greater energy potential. For example, the study revealed a five-fold increase in energy conductivity in indigo-treated water vs. the control water.[1] This is merely one example of a rather simple study, the likes of which have been similarly performed by several other researchers. This particular study is interesting in its separation and comparison of the different effects that the different chakra/spectrum colors had on the properties of the water, as well as its comparison to an ancient healing tradition which used water exposed to direct sunlight that was filtered through colored glass as a therapeutic modality.

From a holistic standpoint, however, it seems somewhat emblematic of some of the basic problems with the approach of modern Western science in these areas of research. A holistic perspective takes a wider look at the influencing factors, and evaluates all of the variables involved for their potential effect on the outcome. The water used was distilled water, sourced from plastic bottles, which is also called 'dead' water, lacking the trace minerals occurring in nature and important for the structuring capacities of water, compromising the integrity of the water (which is already compromised from the plastic bottles in which it was sourced). The light entering the water is not just colored by the cellophane exterior, which may or may not be the specific resonant

1. Cohly HHP, Panja A, Reno WL, III, Obenhuber D, Koelle MS, Das SK, Angel MF, Rao MR. Evidence for Alteration in Chemical and Physical Properties of Water and Modulation of its Biological Functions by Sunlight Transmitted through Color Ranges of the Visible Spectrum – A Novel Study. *International Journal of Environmental Research and Public Health.* 2005; 2(2), 219-227.

harmonic frequency of its color most beneficial and supportive for life (as 'red' represents a band of the electromagnetic spectrum, ranging from near black to near orange). Rather, the sunlight entering the water has passed first through *cellophane* – which, while it is encoded with information of a particular color, also carries the information of its material make-up, which is a rather unnatural form of plastic. Because the water is capable of recognizing and storing *all* of this information – the specific frequency of 'red', mutated by the unnatural structure of plastic cellophane, affected additionally by the plastic from the bottle, as well as any other information to which it was exposed (including the consciousness of the researchers, influenced, for example, by things such as their favorite color, or the emotional response stimulated by certain colors), this type of study is probably not as revealing as it could be.

Both NASA and the U.S. military have been involved with light therapy treatments for decades, and employ its use in treating both astronauts and military personnel. The effects of light on cellular function and accelerated healing having been well documented, particularly in dermatology and in treating seasonal affective disorder. Additional research investigating the effect that various light frequencies from low-level lasers have on certain cellular systems has been ongoing for several years, and researchers have been able to stimulate a variety of cellular responses using different frequencies of light. These include electron transport, adenosine triphosphate (ATP) nitric oxide release, increases in blood flow and reactive oxygen species, as well as the activation of diverse signaling pathways and stem cells. It has also been found effective for treating scarring, wrinkles, burns, and inflammatory conditions such as psoriasis.[2]

What seems to be the result of these two areas of study – the utilization of different light frequencies (colors) to affect health and cellular function, and the study of different light frequencies (colors) on the properties of water – is that light affects the structure and pattern of water in different ways, and the result is what is observed in the effectiveness of light therapies on various diseases, healing acceleration, and cellular activity. And yet while light therapies are effective in effecting the structure of cellular fluids, the frequency patterns and information of specific colors in such therapy methods are largely insufficient to raise the level of crystallographic patterns of the bio-waters to such a degree as to truly cure the root causes of disease and illness, and fully support the body against accelerated aging – or even stop the aging process altogether via non-entropic structural integrity of the DNA and cellular waters. Still, light therapies are an incredibly non-invasive way to affect our health, and we will undoubtedly continue to see development and growth in our therapeutic light technologies and their ability to target the structure of our bio-waters.

2. Asheesh Gupta et al. Low-Level Laser (Light) Therapy (LLT) in Skin: Stimulating, Healing, Restoring. *Seminars in Cutaneous Medicine and Surgery.* March 2013; 32:41-52.

# CHAPTER 24

# SOUND

---

*You are a digital, bio-holographic, precipitation, crystallization, miraculous manifestation, of Divine frequency vibrations, coming out of Water. Get it? You are the music, echoing universally and eternally hydro-sonically.*
~DR. LEONARD HOROWITZ, D.M.D., M.A., M.P.H, D.N.M.
RESEARCHER, AUTHOR, HUMANITARIAN

Sound, much like light, is also known for generating strong effects on the structure of water. Photographic work of ice crystals shows the different effects that various types of music has on the crystallographic patterns of ice crystals, and sound-treated water has had successful results when used to treat various diseases, ailments, and mental disorders, or when employed to stimulate consciousness, relaxation, or meditation. Sound evokes emotion, triggers changes in our consciousness, mood, and even our health. The different patterns and geometries generated by various frequencies of sound can be seen in the popular cymatics experiments (cymatics: the study of visible sound and vibration), wherein a specific note of vibration is played to a platform of scattered sand, which bounces and moves in response to the vibration, creating different designs and geometric formations on the plate. The entire pattern and picture created by the sand on the plate can change in response to even the slightest change in pitch or tone. Here also we see the water-structuring aspects of toning, drumming, mantras, and chanting. Today, there are many people who practice sacred toning (or the singing and/ or repeating of certain notes and sounds) to affect health, consciousness, and wellness. It has been described by some Ayurvedic and Buddhist practitioners that to repeat a mantra, sound, or word, is to build the energy of that sound until it reverberates and vibrates through your entire being, until it has generated a 'standing-wave' field in and around the body – which in this case can be thought of as a resounding, reverberating echo that does not dissipate but rather continues to resonate within your being ('standing-wave' as opposed to traveling wave – it vibrates in place, rather than 'travels', these are also termed 'scalar waves'). In these traditions, integrating the pattern of a specific mantra or word (*Om*, for example) permanently into the structure of the bio-waters and its auric and bio-energetic systems as that resonating resounding standing wave, can take years of intense repetition and mental training. So while sound, like light, is an effective method of providing structural information to a system, it also is generally insufficient alone in establishing and providing the intricately complex crystallographic patterns required by the cellular systems for true longevity and health, and is rather another piece of the holistic puzzle.

# CHAPTER 25

# MAGNETISM

---

*The property ordinarily called magnetism, is, in reality, a
peculiar activity in the surrounding ether, known technically
as magnetic flux... it is that of the ether in translatory
motion... in a magnet, ether is actually streaming out from the
north-seeking pole and re-entering at the south-seeking pole.*
~W.J. JOHNSTON
ELECTRICAL WORLD: VOLUME 24

Magnetism is an interesting force in the realm of water
and health, particularly as it relates to theories of
magneto-electric energy and the connection with subtle
energies of healers and consciousness, as observed in the
similarities of healer-treated water and magnetically-
treated water. Water displays a reaction to magnetism
and reacts differently, exhibiting different structural
patterns, based on the type of magnetic information to
which it is exposed (i.e. strength of magnetism, type of
magnetic material used, north pole vs. south pole, vs.
mixed pole exposure, etc.). This phenomena has long

found practical application in steam boilers, where water
is exposed to a magnetic field and thus becomes less hard
and produces less scale than ordinary water. Water
treated by magnets also shows an increase in surface
tension, viscosity, and electrical conductivity, and affects
the behavior and vital activity of living organisms.
Magnetically treated water accelerates the growth of
seedlings and plants, and experiments with mice have
shown that in "the animals [that] were given intravenous
injections of water which had been exposed to a magnetic
field…there was increased urination in 63% of the cases
in comparison to animals which had received an injection
of ordinary water."[1]

Different *types* of magnetism generate different effects
in water, which indicates that different types and levels
of magnetism cause different structural arrangements in
water. The implication here is that there is *pattern
differentiation within various magnetic fields* – in other
words, magnetic fields generate or affect the patterns of
information within their field in an exacting way to the
specific type of magnetic information, much in the same
way that electromagnetic waves generate patterns of
information within their fractal 'wave-forms' and
frequencies. In the field of subtle energy, magnets and
magnetism are often referred to as "ether" pumps, or
subtle energy pumps, for their ability to interact with
and drive subtle energy, demonstrated in the effects of
magnetism on water and bio-energetic systems. In a
magnet, subtle energy (which is highly magnetic in
nature) streams out from the north-seeking pole, while it

1. Cope, Freeman W. "Magnetoelectric charge states of matter-energy. A
second approximation." *Journal of Physiology Chemistry & Physics.* 12, (1980).
337-341.

enters (or re-enters) through the south-seeking pole in a vortexing toroidal field.[2]

We see further implications of pattern differentiation within magnetic fields in plant growth response, as magnetic fields of relatively low intensity has been found to be effective in stimulating or initiating plant growth responses. Exposing seeds, seedlings, and plants to magnetic fields indicate improved water uptake, seedling length, germination rates, seedling length, fresh weights, and plant vigor.[3] Tested seeds have been found to germinate faster and grow more when they were placed in a certain position relative to the magnetic field, specifically when they were oriented longitudinally parallel to the lines of force.[4] There is no lack of research into the effects of magnetic fields on plant growth: Pretreatment of cumin seeds (called "magnetopriming") has demonstrated faster germination and growth, increase in volatile oils and cumin seeds post maturity, and an increase in chlorophyll content.[5] Vertical magnetic fields have also demonstrated significant increases in total fresh shoot weights and fresh root weights, and research suggests that the promotion of cell elongation under low magnetic fields may correlate to an increase of osmotic pressure in the cells. Most interesting,

2. Johnston, W.J. *Electrical World, Volume 24.* Electrical Engineering, 1894.

3. Maffei ME Magnetic field effects on plant growth, development, and evolution. *Front. Plant Sci.* 2014; 5:445. doi: 10.3389/fpls.2014.00445

4. Pittman, UJ. Magnetism and Plant Growth: Effect on Germination and Early Growth of Cereal Seeds. *Canadian Journal of Plant Science.* 1963; 43(4): 513-518.

5. Jamshid Razmjoo & Sara Alinian. Influence of Magnetopriming on Germination, Growth, Physiology, Oil and Essential Contents of Cumin. *Electromagnetic Biology and Medicine.* 2017: 36:4, 325-329. DOI: 10.1080/15368378.2017.1373661

perhaps, is the indication that mitochondria are the most sensitive organelle to low magnetic field treatments, which increase their size and relative volume in response.[6]

Magnetic therapies in health care are widely successful, and are now being integrated into medical centers and hospitals in the form of Transcranial Magnetic Stimulation (TMS) therapy, sometimes costing more than $10,000 per treatment. Magnetic bracelets, knee pads, mattress toppers, chair pads, and various other forms of magnetic therapy devices are becoming more and more popular as people experience relief from pain, arthritis, and numerous chronic and acute ailments, including degenerative disc disease and cancer. The body, however, is most responsive to low-level magnetic fields, and the quality and type of magnetic material and induction is important. Many people with chronic diseases such as pain and arthritis experience a certain degree of initial relief from using magnetic forms of therapy, however the relief often seems to plateau at some point and never fully realize a 'cure' or full relief of symptoms or dis-ease. So while magnets and magnetism have a strong effect on water and health, much like light and sound, again it is insufficient on it's own to bring about a true evolution of the body's system back to harmony or an even higher order of function. Certainly, however, the research into plant science demonstrates the influential effect magnetic fields can have on water and biological processes of life and health, showing us how magnetism is yet another piece of a holistic approach to water restructuring.

6. Maffei, ME. 2014.

# CHAPTER 26

# VORTEXING

---

*Spirals are a basic form of motion in Nature... the vortex [is] the principle creative movement system in the Universe... from the tornado to plant growth, it is nature's mechanism for transforming energy from one level to another.*
~ALICK BARTHOLOMEW
AUTHOR: WRITING ABOUT VIKTOR
SCHAUBERGER

One of Nature's most primary and principle forces is the power of a vortex. Vortices or vortexes are seen everywhere in nature – in whirlpools and water movements, tornadoes, hurricanes, plants, seashells, implosions, our venous system, and galaxies. It has been found to have a powerful effect on water, capable of causing an increase in structure that can result in purification, when properly applied. Most of our information regarding water and vortex action comes from the work of Viktor Schauberger, who developed theories of Implosion principles based on his observations and study of the vortices occurring in naturally flowing water and weather patterns. Through the research and development of these theories, he was able to produce spring-quality water, as well as generate considerable energy sources. Dr. Marcel Vogel also used vortex principles during his water structuring methods, described in the following section. There are multiple devices being sold on the market to vortex water and thus improve its quality, and some are effective to a degree – though much more effective when used in conjunction with other methods such as sound, crystals, and/or magnetism. Of course, when we consider the water in our bodies, vortex principles are not necessarily applicable as a method of treatment,p as the natural vortex methods of our physical systems should not necessarily be stimulated outside of their natural state. Vortex principles will be important to apply in the development of various external water-structuring units, and the work of Viktor Schauberger and others should be more fully investigated for their structuring potentials. Gratefully, there are some phenomenal authors who have covered Viktor Schauberger's work in great detail, such as Callum Coats and Alick Bartholomew. For further reading on Viktor Schauberger, I highly recommend *Living Energies* by Callum Coats, or Alick Bartholomew's book *Hidden Nature: The Startling Insights of Viktor Schauberger.*

CHAPTER 27

# CRYSTALS AND MINERALS

Crystals and minerals are the most abundant material on earth, while water is the most abundant substance. They have been used for water structuring purposes and their effects on subtle energy since antiquity, revered by humanity for all of time, all across the world. The remnants of our historical appreciation for crystals and gems are visible in our ancient scriptures, imagery, and ruins, permeating traditions, legends, and cultures. Gems and various types of crystals are found in nearly every dig of any past civilizations and their remains, used for sacred and religious purposes as well as medicinal and healing in virtually every tradition in history. Ancient China and Traditional Chinese Medicine, ancient India and Ayurvedic medicine, Traditional Tibetan Medicine, Native American traditions, aboriginals and indigenous peoples, Judeo-Christians, the nation of Islam, ancient Egypt, the Roman Empire, ancient Greece, ancient Babylonia – if there is a tradition, it more than likely incorporated crystals into its practice or legends, and it may be because of the energy patterns of crystals and their effects on water, and thus their effects on consciousness, spirit, and health.

They have been considered a source of mystery and power for centuries, ascribed to the realms of oracles and prophets, sorcerers and magicians, emperors and kings. Besides the common description of the throne of God being associated with various types of crystals and precious materials, and the description in Revelations in the New Testament of the New Age being a type of crystal city, there is also general sense among many Christians and Biblical scholars that the rod of Moses and Aaron was or had on it some type of crystal. Specific crystals were inlaid on the breastplate of Aaron, as was the mysterious *Urim* and *Thummim* of Old Testament literature, which were some type (or types) of objects (likely crystals) with very interesting properties. One of the ways these were employed was in the practice of divination, i.e. for testing subtle energy, or receiving yes or no answers to specific questions by using tools that interact with the subtle energy and magneto-electric fields, responding in a way that can be interpreted for further meaning. This process is sometimes referred to as 'dowsing', which is a practice not limited to finding water sources but rather can be an effective way of discerning information and changes in subtle energy fields, a practice still used today by many to locate underground sources of water, including public utility officials in the UK. In Islam, there is the mysterious and sacred 'black stone', which has been set inside of the Holy Temple at Mecca. It is said that the missing capstones on the Great Pyramids were crystal, and of course there is the heavy use of crystals and crystal technologies in Plato's description of Atlantis.

It is through the study of crystals that we learned geometry, sacred and repeating pattern formation, and fundamental lessons of physics and computer processing. Studying how light refracts and moves through various crystal shapes, and how different types of energy are transmuted from one form to another – such as mechanical pressure to electricity in the piezoelectric property of quartz – is how we have been able to advance our knowledge of science and technology to the level we experience today. And it is not just our past and our present science that is heavily rooted in crystals, it is also our future. Today, our entire technological age is dependent on the use and incorporation of crystals, and they have in their own right defined our very era.

As liquid crystalline water is in the same family of atomic structures as solid-state crystals (i.e. crystallographic patterns), it comes as no surprise that crystals have a strong effect on the structure of water. Operating on the same geometric principles of molecular formations, liquid crystalline water and solid-state crystals have a natural type of resonance. Not coherent resonance, necessarily, but resonance enough to allow a level of information transfer and processing. And because the energy and electromagnetic waves emitting from crystals are fractalized with their information – including that of their geometric pattern formation – water is able to receive and process this information, reflected in its adjusted structure, changes in properties, and increased bio-availability after exposure to certain types and cuts of crystals. As animals can easily tell the difference between structured water and bulk, non-structured, or de-structured water, so too do people know the difference, particularly those who have trained their awareness and sensitivities as our ancestors did.

Filtering water through crystals and minerals does wonders for its quality and structure. Some crystals are better known for their actions on water when filtered, for example magnetite (a paramagnetic mineral form of iron ore) and shungite (a mineral from Russia, composed of 30-98% carbon, depending on quality). Shungite has been used in medical treatment since the early 18th century, was used by Peter the Great in the first Russian spa, and is also used for providing purified water for the Russian army. As we mentioned earlier, the anti-bacterial properties of shungite have been confirmed by modern testing, and shungite water filtration has been observed to clean water of various chlorine compounds and fluoride, as well as remove heavy metals, increase levels of potassium and anti-oxidant power, and purify almost all organic compounds, including pesticides, bacteria, and harmful microorganisms, through its structuring properties.[1] These changes in the water's structure are also responsible for shungite water's reputed ability to aid with allergies, through an antihistamine effect, relieve inflammation and symptoms of chronic fatigue, depression, trauma, common colds, asthma, diabetes, pancreatic, liver, kidney, or gall-bladder issues, burns, acne, arthritis, etc. Shungite has a unique crystalline structure, which includes a heavy carbon base and the only known natural source of fullerenes on Earth (with the exception of a few meteorites).[2] Fullerenes are full carbon molecules which can act as hollow cages, resonate in the far infrared spectrum with all forms of living matter, and are thought to be connected with the generation of life. The structural composition of shungite

1. Selinus O., Finkelman R.B. and Centeno, J.A. Medical Geology: A Regional Synthesis. Springer, 2010.
2. Dagani, Ron. Fullerenes in Nature: C60 and C70 found in ancient Russian Rock. *Chemical Engineering News.* 1992; 70(28): 6. DOI: 10.1021/cen-v070n028.p006

also includes the likely presence of "Buckminster-fullerenes" or "buckyballs" as well, which are specific sphere shaped fullerene molecules. It is theorized that the specific fullerene structures within shungite lend towards its ability to aid in purification with optimal micro-mineral composition and a highly bio-available and beneficial structure. In a similar fashion, magnetite filtration processes have been observed to increase the atomic hydrogen and oxygen levels in water, cause purification, and express other structurally related changes.

As water moves over and around multiple stones and structures, it undergoes something called "structural interface activity", something that happens naturally in our environment as water is filtered up through layers of minerals in the case of erupting springs, or over multiple rocks and movements as it channels its way back to the sea. As water comes into contact with and moves around different minerals, it not only incorporates traces of these minerals into it's composition, it also uses them to increase its structure. Certain marketers have taken advantage of this process using something as basic as marbles or glass balls – something that can be created at home for a fraction of the price in a DIY fashion, to affect the structure of your water to a minimal degree. Others use specific minerals and stones to remineralize drinking water, with varying degrees of effectiveness. For more information on DIY options, or the remineralizing systems I use and recommend, please see the Resources section and the end of this book.

The most incredible development of crystals for the use of structuring water came from the work of the great crystallographer, the father of structured water science, and one of the most prolific inventors of our time, the previously mentioned Dr. Marcel Vogel. Retiring from nearly 30 years with IBM after developing numerous patents as one of their most valuable researchers, Dr. Vogel established a research institute fully equipped with donations from his former employer. It was here that Dr. Marcel Vogel embarked on his quest to further investigate the link between crystals and consciousness. Dr. Vogel understood several important facts about crystals and water that had been either previously ignored or were as yet undiscovered. First, he recognized that quartz crystals have a special relationship with consciousness and subtle energy, in that quartz causes the *amplification* and storage of subtle energies. This relationship is capable of causing changes within the structure of the quartz itself in response to the subtle energetic stimuli. This is the result of an effective encoding of information, usually referred to as the 'programming' or 'tuning' of the crystal (as in tuning to a particular frequency). It was this type of revelation that allowed for the development of using crystals as information storage, a fact previously referenced in the numerous holographic images already successfully stored in 'crystal databases.'

Also important was Dr. Vogel's understanding of how to *clear* the programming absorbed by the quartz, using a bulk de-magnetizer. In terms of subtle energy, quartz is an *indiscriminate* amplifier and database. It does not discern against negative energies and consciousness, rather it will amplify and store that information as well, information that is essentially highly entropic and causes a de-structuring effect rather than improving towards a non-entropic, or syntropic, structure. It can pick up this information from the consciousness and energetic fields of both people and the environment, whether it is in the form of negative thought patterns, both conscious and subconscious, harmful artificial electromagnetic frequencies permeating the airspace, or otherwise damaging, non-life supporting, and entropic energy sources. Recall that subtle-energies are energies outside of our perceivable spectrum (including consciousness), and that they are likely to be magneto-electric rather than electro-magnetic. Being strongly magnetic in nature, Dr. Vogel's approach to clearing the information with a de-magnetizer (which erases magnetic encoding) was both sound theory and a necessary protocol. He recognized not only the infinite amount of potential information storage within a single crystal, but also the implications of indiscriminate energetic amplification and the potential effects on an individual from un-intentional information storage (i.e. harmful and artificial EMF's and EMR's in an environment, negative thought patterns, etc.).

Dr. Vogel also understood that the *shape* of the quartz crystal affected its ability to focus, amplify, cohere, and transmit energy. Earlier when discussing coherence we used the example of specifically cut rubies cohering light waves into a resonantly integrated stream of coherency, known as a laser. Thus, Dr. Vogel recognized that quartz could be cut into a specific shape to operate on the same coherence and transmission properties of rubies, with the added effect of the amplification provided by the structure of the quartz. Additionally, he recognized that quartz crystal, made of silicon dioxide ($SiO_2$), had a unique structural compatibility with water, in that they are both hexagonal and essentially "fit together", and that this has profound implications on the ability of a properly cut quartz crystal to affect the molecular structure of water and water-based liquids. When he finally established the proper crystal shape to amplify, cohere, and transmit subtle energy, he discovered that *the specifically cut quartz crystal resonated at the same frequency of water,* as established through frequency evaluations using the most advanced radionics equipment known to man even today, the Omega 5. This frequency resonance indicated the highest level of coherence, and thus a high amount of resonant information transfer between the specifically cut crystal and water.

Resonant information transfer was the key, and this allowed Marcel to operate in an entire new world of structuring water. With specifically cut quartz crystals, he was able to take energies operating on the subtle energy and magneto-electric spectrum and transmit them as a coherently patterned 'waveform' in resonant transmission to water. Coherent resonance, as we recall, allows for the greatest amount of information transfer. When specific intentions, consciousness, and subtle energies were stored in and passed through the molecular structure of the quartz, they were amplified and transmitted to water with full integrity.

The process of transmitting information from one system to another can be thought of as a dialogue, or a translation. Information from one system, in the language of its specific fractal–patterned energy signature, must be translated by another system in order to be processed by that system as information, and in order for the receiving system to initiate the proper response. Language here is an appropriate metaphor – consider twins, who can resonate so well together they appear to communicate with just thought, or even act as a single entity in perfect synchronization; as compared to translating a completely foreign language, in which there is often great meaning lost in translation, when translation is even possible. With perfect resonance, there is no loss in translation during information transmission, reception, decoding, processing, or response.

Dr. Vogel, having developed specifically cut quartz crystals that resonated at the same frequency of pristine water, was thus able to transfer the amplified and cohered subtle energy information of consciousness, energy, and intentional programming (recall the infinite amount of information storage potential within single crystals) to the water with full integrity, allowing for the greatest amount of correct and 'in phase' information transfer. This was extremely important. Once able to store consciousness and intentional information into the quartz, which is encoded within its molecular structure as specific patterns of information, coherent resonance between the frequencies of the quartz and water allowed the highest amount of information transfer. The information now structurally encoded into the quartz could be transferred to the water, which in turn encoded this information into its structural arrangement. This is how Dr. Vogel became the first father of structured water science, using specifically cut quartz crystals to affect the molecular structure of water, operating within the realm of subtle energy and magneto-electricity. Using these specifically cut quartz crystals, Dr. Vogel found he could effectively change the properties of water, causing the expressions of its liquid crystalline state and dynamic changes in the formation of its crystallographic patterns.

Through extensive study and experimentation, Dr. Vogel came to establish protocols for the structuring of fluids to affect their preservation rate and integrity using the specifically cut crystal he created, referred to today as a "Vogel" crystal, or "Vogel-cut". His protocols involved the use of the electromagnetic field generated by the movement of water, vortexing the water around specifically programmed and cut quartz crystals. Using these methods, he was able to demonstrate the improved structure of juices and milk, through a dramatic prolonging of shelf life. He also demonstrated the rapid aging of a newly created wine – indicating that the structural changes that make aged wine much more refined and palatable had occurred through Marcel Vogel's structuring process using his cut quartz crystals. These types of results were astounding, and demonstrated concepts about the structure of water that were beyond nearly all the scientists of his time. Just as today the researchers at Princeton are investigating the potentials for structuring water for the preservation of pharmaceutical drugs, so Dr. Vogel was successfully and dramatically extending the preservation of milk and juices 20 years before their preservation theories. And in the wine industry, the ability to rapidly age wine without compromising the integrity of the flavor and texture is a much sought after advantage. More important than extending the shelf life of milk or juice, or rapidly aging wine, however, was the "Vogel" crystal's ability to work as a tool for healing.

Programming the quartz with intention and consciousness, using mental training and specific breathing techniques and protocols, Dr. Vogel and those he trained were able to induce changes into the physical and energetic systems of an individual for healing through affecting the structure of the body's water. By establishing resonance between the cut and programmed (or 'tuned') crystal itself and the water in the individual, he was able to convey highly intentional consciousness energy that could be used by the bio-energetic body for healing. Dr. Vogel and his research team performed incredible healing sessions, surprising doctors and patients alike with their ability to alleviate pain and relieve and heal multiple types of disorders and diseases.

Dr. Vogel's techniques were heavily dependent upon three things – the proper methods for faceting the specifically cut crystal, the 'charge' or 'programming' that one was able to invoke into the quartz itself, and the trained consciousness of the healer. Although his results were phenomenal, and the widespread potential applications very promising, Dr. Vogel knew that the dependence upon these three factors was an incredible challenge, both in sharing his technology with the world and expanding the possibilities for other applications. His technique for cutting a proper Vogel-cut crystal was based on more than just the angles of the facets or the length and width ratios of the crystal; it was also dependent upon the consciousness and subtle energy influences during the cutting process. Dr. Vogel demonstrated this with a comparative exercise – after providing the proper dimensional specifications to highly trained crystal workers, he compared both of them using the Omega 5. Although the other crystal was physically cut exactly the same as Marcel Vogel's, it still failed to vibrate at a harmonic frequency to water. Marcel's crystal, of course, did. He had greatly enhanced his conscious awareness and mental abilities through meditative, spiritual, and intellectual training, and had established specific methods for operating harmoniously with the responsive nature of quartz. This allowed him to achieve a remarkably high level of information storage using conscious intention alone, as well as to direct those energies through the crystal appropriately for healing. Unfortunately, very few people, if any, have the mental training and skill that Marcel had for working with quartz.

It is for this reason that he performed numerous training sessions and classes, created and programmed numerous crystals before his passing, and laid the groundwork for further research and development through his instruction and legacy. Before his early passing, he charged fellow scientists and researchers to continue to advance his work, recognizing the supreme implications of water-resonant information transfer via specifically cut quartz crystals. Sadly, his work has largely been misunderstood or capitalized on by unethical and unreliable marketers. Buyer beware! If you would like to be connected with a *reputable* source, please check the Resources at the end of this book.

# CHAPTER 28

# CONSCIOUSNESS

---

*You are not a drop in the ocean.*
*You are the entire ocean, in a drop.*
~RUMI

Water's high responsiveness to consciousness is a fact that may feel a bit redundant at this point, but as it is another primary method of structuring it is a necessary one to include in this section. Consciousness does amazing things to water, and water does amazing things to consciousness. Simply being *around* water has a powerful effect on our physical and mental well-being. Wallace Nichols, author of Blue Mind, put it this way: "The ocean and wild waterways are a wellspring of happiness and relaxation, sociality and romance, peace and freedom, play and creativity, learning and memory, innovation and insight, elation and nostalgia, confidence and solitude, wonder and awe, empathy and compassion, reverence and beauty – and help manage trauma, anxiety, sleep, autism, addiction, fitness, attention/focus, stress, grief, PTSD, build personal resilience...Being on, in, and near water can be among the most cost-effective was of reducing stress and anxiety." He goes on to say that the "realization of the full range and potential magnitude of ecological, economic, physical, intrinsic, and emotional values of wild places requires us to understand, appreciate, maintain, and improve the integrity and purity of one of our most vital of medicines – water."[1]

It can be logically assumed that water's high responsiveness to consciousness and the high responsiveness of consciousness to water reflects a level of resonance between the two. We have already examined the incredible connection between water and consciousness and explored the relationship between consciousness and water, wherein it appears that consciousness is actually energetic information stored in the molecular structure of the water inside of our bodies, and this resonance allows consciousness (energetic information stored in our bio-waters) to be transferred to water (where it also is stored as energetic information) with incredible coherence, and virtually no loss of information during transfer.

So if our consciousness is in coherent resonance with water, why not just mentally structure all of the water to which we are exposed, as well as all of the water inside of our bodies? Obviously it is not that simple. Structuring water with consciousness is not as easy as it seems, particularly when one considers the level of consciousness which most people experience. The average attention span is approximately 6 seconds. Having total focus and concentration to direct all of your mental faculties at a single, undistracted task and intention is something that usually takes extensive training, akin to the trainings of monks or 'Chi masters' (masters of subtle energy and Chi or Qi, a.k.a. 'life-force',

---

1. Nichols, Wallace J. *Blue Mind: The Surprising Science That Shows How Being Near, In, On, or Under Water Can Make You Happier, Healthier, More Connected, and Better at What You Do.* Back Bay Books. 2015.

i.e. Qi-gong masters). And in a world where our level of focused consciousness is being constantly attacked and bombarded by our media, EMF pollution, and the overall toxicity of our food, water, and air supply, to rely on consciousness alone for structuring external water sources is terribly insufficient. Using consciousness to structure the bio-waters is even more challenging, since the de-structuring that has occurred is intimately linked to the level of consciousness it has and is experiencing. Neuro-linguistic programming (NLP), positive thinking, mantras, meditations, mindfulness, and psychology methods are just a few examples of current consciousness practices whose unrecognized goal is actually a re-structuring of bio-waters, to in turn affect the physical, mental, and energetic systems through their role in the bio-feedback loop. As our level of consciousness is limited by the structure of our water, and the structure of our water is in turn limited by our level of consciousness, interceding in this bio-feedback loop is difficult and often requires aids and tools to assist us. Making sure that the water we are putting into our bodies is free of contaminants, well mineralized, and structured (or, at the very least, not de-structured) also aids our body in raising our level of consciousness (see Resources for recommendations on drinking water or bio-water structuring tools). Regular mindfulness practices are essential, as is building support for these practices in your daily life, whether from participating in a group, using an app or meditation program, or developing yoga or mindfulness exercise practices.

CHAPTER 29

# NATURE

---

*If there is magic on this planet,*
*it is contained in Water.*
~LOREN EISLEY
SCIENCE WRITER

As Life is dependent upon the complex structure of water, we need only look to see Nature's water structuring processes all around us. The Earth structures water through intense mineral filtering and composition – in fact, you will never find water features in nature that doesn't have some type of mineral composition and trace elements, whether it's calcium, magnesium, silica, manganese, germanium, etc. The natural occurring mineral filtration processes in nature are an essential aspect of providing crystalline structures to the water and the minerals necessary for biological life. It structures its water with sunlight, moonlight, and the lights of the planets and stars in the cosmos of the night sky. The sounds of the Earth structure her waters; as well as its birds, bees, and animal life, the wind blowing through the trees, the sounds of thunder and clouds rolling overhead. Nature structures the waters of the Earth every time it processes through the natural water cycle of evaporation, condensation, and precipitation, and every time it travels a natural, winding, or curving path along its nutrient rich earth before flowing back to the sea. It structures water with the frequencies of the Schumann Resonance and the Earth's electromagnetic field. It structures water with subtle energy charging; the consciousness of the organisms in their ecosystems, the consciousness of the planet, and through electromagnetic ley lines, vortexes, and nodal points located on the Earth. These electromagnetic ley lines represent a type of meridian system on the Earth, where electromagnetism and subtle energy condense and cycle through various channels on the Earth. Points where these channels intersect are called vortex points, or nodal points, creating a spinning wheel of energy where the various lines cross. Water located along these ley lines and at different vortex sites is highly structured and is often associated with holy sites and sacred water sources, or connected to some miraculous event(s) representing an increase in subtle energy and consciousness.

But despite this perfectly designed system of cycling, purifying, mineralizing, and re-structuring the waters on the planet, we still find ourselves at a point where clean water can be hard enough to find, much less highly structured water. The level of pollution experienced by the planet is at a level never before seen in human history, and its water structuring system stands little chance against the "electro-smog" of high artificial electromagnetic frequencies bombarding and permeating the airs around us, the contamination of our groundwater, rivers, lakes, and seas by industrial pollutants, the chaotic consciousness and energetic imbalances of our communities and cities, and the ever-increasing heavy metals and other contaminants being released into our atmosphere on a daily basis in the form of chem-trails (the lingering visible trails left by jet airplanes, not to be confused with con-trails, the trails of water and ice that dissipate rather quickly, but rather jet streams that contain chemical toxins such as aluminum and barium compounds which leave long and persistent trails, once denied as the subject of conspiracy theories and now generally acknowledged), the systemic toxicity of disinfecting agents and byproducts, microplastics, and radioactive isotopes, coupled by massively failing infrastructure and public health officials who more often then not are beholden to industry demands to keep maximum contaminant levels higher than they should be.

While highly structured waters at one point existed all over the Earth, we now find them in remote and hard to find areas in mountainous or glacial regions, and even then we can no longer find any source of water, anywhere in the world, which has not been contaminated with PCB's or pharmaceuticals. The systemic pollution we have caused on our planet has penetrated even our Earth's water cycle, where the pollutants are caught up, as it were, reaching remote areas so far from man they never should have been contaminated. And while simply spending time in Nature and exposing oneself to the natural forms of light, sound, energy, and frequencies of our natural environment can have amazing effects and is incredibly therapeutic, both consciously and physically, when it comes to structuring the waters inside of the body, simply spending time in Nature is such a gentle and non-invasive structuring method that it is extremely unlikely to be able to penetrate the consciousness of most people to such a degree as to raise the level of molecular complexity high enough to overcome cancers, heart disease, diabetes, HIV, or aging.

When the integrity of our tap water is virtually non-existent, a plethora of carcinogens disguised as safe drinking water, and our bottled water may even be worse, when a lifetime of exposure to toxicity and poor water quality has left our bio-waters in worse form than they should be, we turn again to Nature. What is necessary for clean, quality, life promoting water, and how do we maintain our own body's structure? Nature starts with water that is not contaminated with carcinogens, and has intricate purification and remineralization systems. So too do we need a complete purification of our drinking water, followed by a spectrum of remineralization – not just some cheap filter on a fridge and a pH buffer of bicarbonate or calcium, but a high integrity, intense purification system followed by full spectrum remineralization. Natural light, music and sound, rhythmic movement, low level magnetic fields, subtle energy exposure, positive intention and consciousness – these are all Nature's methods of maintaining the health of her source of Life, and the force which sustains it. So too do we need time in natural light (and away from artificial light), to immerse ourselves in music, sound, and rhythmic movements, to practice subtle energy exercises or modalities such as acupuncture and reiki, and to spend time developing control and intention with our consciousness by spending time in nature, spending time near *water*, building positive and harmonious relationships with our environment and others in it, and practicing meditation, intentional breathing, or focused exercises such as yoga. While the focus of therapies targeted at restructuring the body's water may focus on water resonance or crystal patterns, it is important to recognize that *water* is *water resonant,* and the Earth has an incredible ability to transform us through our connection with Nature.

# PART VI

# THE ANSWER TO
# THE QUESTION

CHAPTER 30

# HOW TO AFFECT THE STRUCTURE OF THE CELLULAR FLUIDS

Having seen the various methods employed by Nature and man to structure water, we quickly realize the inadequacies of these methods when discussing the re-structuring of the bio-water system. The molecular structures of the waters in our bodies and the crystallographic patterns formed by them are *incredibly* complex. The molecules are so small, so elaborately combined and multi-dimensionally intricate, and are ever changing in response to the needs of the physical body and the energetic and consciousness stimuli to which it is exposed. Thus we realize that the crystallographic pattern information of our bio-waters requires fractal and infinitely complex arrangements that support its dynamic and ever changing need.

Sound, light, magnetism, vortex action, consciousness, and generally speaking, even crystals, are all effective ways of altering the structure of water to a certain degree, but these methods are generally incomplete and insufficient – whether used alone or in conjunction – particularly as it applies to bio-waters. Each modality, separate or together, does not provide the intricate crystallographic patterns needed by the multi-dimensional complex ordering of our bio-waters. To do this, we need the actual crystallographic patterns and complex combinations of different geometries. We find this information expressed in the different crystallographic patterns of the multiple crystals, gems, and minerals so abundant in and on the Earth, used for centuries for various water and healing practices. Crystals, as we have seen, are an expression of a particular pattern of geometric arrangement of information, and through combining multiple groups of crystals, each expressing different pattern arrangements, we are able to arrive at the level of complex crystallographic patterns required by the water in our bodies.

In order to use these patters to affect the molecular structure of the bio-waters, we need a way to combine these various groups of crystals and minerals in an integrated way, fitting them together within each other in nested, 'in-phase', coherent harmonious patterns of information. Then, we need to take this harmonious, complex combination of crystallographic patterns and coherently transmit the information of their structural arrangements in a way that will be resonantly received by the body's water and bio-energetic systems. This type of energy transference – one that is in resonant coherence with the body's water and bio-energetic systems, in order to be resonantly received and coherently processed – involves working the subtle energy spectrum, i.e. in the realm of magneto-electricity, subtle energy vortex centers, meridian lines, etc. This is no small task, and is most certainly at least two-fold: harmonically and coherently nesting the pattern information of multiple crystallographic forms, and inducing this complex combination into the waters of the body in a way that it will be correctly received and processed, i.e. in resonance.

Operating in the field of subtle energy (as our bio-waters do in their intimate connection with consciousness) requires a harmonious working with the body's subtle energy system, recognizing the needs and mechanics of its crystallographic patterns, bio-energetic systems, and their corresponding biofeedback loops. Perhaps this is why no scientist has every truly answered Dr. Gyorgi's call, as Western science has yet to really accept the subtle energy systems described by the Chinese and Ayurvedic traditions of chakras and meridians, despite the overwhelming evidence supporting their existence.

Throughout this research, we continue to arrive at what seemed to be the true key to health, longevity, and the evolution of consciousness, spirit, and life – affecting the molecular structure of the water and bio-energetic systems towards greater non-entropic forms. By doing so, we establish greater coherence across the entire system, increasing the level of function in the brain, body, and energy field, creating a more efficient, stable, synchronized, and cohered being. As our waters and energy systems are infused with an abundance of the crystallographic pattern information on which they depend to maintain and develop our self-organized system, we begin to see evidence of measurable changes in the bio-energetic systems, as well as measurable changes in thought patterns, perceptions, emotional states, desires, motivations, direction, and all other aspects of self: self-wants, self-needs, self-confidence, self-worth, etc.

The fundamental understanding amongst innumerable researchers, practitioners, and healing modalities is that changes in the physical structure, whether towards health or disease, occur as a result of changes in the bio-energetic system. My research also supports this well-founded theory, a theory that will undoubtedly one day be accepted as fact. But the research also indicates that changes in the molecular structure of the water can precede changes in the bio-energetic system, acting in the feedback loop of energy, water, and the corresponded manifested state of being (whether biological, emotional, or mental) to not only be affected by changes in the bio-energetic system but to also *cause* changes in the bio-energetic system. Following the simultaneous expression of changes in the bio-energetic systems, changes in the physical function and structure appear in appropriate correlation to the manifested state of being as a result of the cascade of changes within the water and bio-energetic systems of the body. The expression of assessable changes in these two states – that of adjustments in the bio-energetic systems and noticeable changes in consciousness – are in reality reflecting the original source of change and effect: the structure of the water in the body.

Thus, recall our discussion on the origination of a *thought* – the same instant that we perceive a thought, we have a simultaneous reaction throughout the entire physical system – immune response, heart rate variability, hormone and bio-chemical triggers and release, electromagnetic fluctuations, etc. Scientists expected that the thought in the brain would *precede* the reactions in the body, rather than occur simultaneously, were puzzled by this and still left asking the question *where does the origination of the thought occur, or come from?* From a structured water perspective, this is exactly what we would expect, and the question posed is quickly answered. The origination of the thought occurs first in structural changes within the body's bio-water system, which is prompted through any one of water's highly responsive conscious, magneto-electric, electro-magnetic, or otherwise energetic stimuli and triggers. In response to the change in structure, the body and the brain react simultaneously as expected. Electrical patterns in the brain are fired in accordance to the structural information and processed as the "thought", changes in the immune system, heart rate variability, blood stream, digestion, hormone and bio-chemical levels, and electromagnetic fluctuations also happen instantaneously in accordance to the structural information, causing the body to exhibit the appropriate response. Thus, the body's physiological response and the brain's linear processing of information are always in complete tandem, because they are both reacting to the structural information change in the bio-water system. Here we begin to truly grasp the importance of the structure of our bio-waters in our biofeedback system, in recognizing its action in stimulating both conscious perception and specific types of thought patterns and mental processing, as well as stimulating a corresponding instantaneous and cascading physical effect and chain reaction. Raising the level of structure in our bio-waters results in greater coherence and better brain function, higher levels of awareness, greater experiences of joy and increased positivity, emotional stability and an improved sense of self-worth, motivation, happiness, and vitality, relief from chronic dehydration and its associated symptoms, greater physical health and wellness, stronger immune system, accelerated healing rates, more efficient digestion, metabolic balance, strengthened and balanced bio-energetic systems, increased longevity, the perception and experience of more meaningful relationships, a greater sense of spirituality, peace, self-reflection, and enhanced creativity, improved abilities to meditate or process larger amounts of information not previously perceived, etc. The list could continue, as humans are complex creatures and express changes within our systems in a variety of ways. Overall, the message is clear: through improving our structure, we can improve ourselves.

# WATER AND THE ETHERS: THE OCEAN OF THE UNIVERSE

## As Above, So Below – and Everywhere in Between

Water is intrinsically connected to the *aether* or *ether,* the common term for the sea of energy within the Universe. This concept can also be discussed in terms of 'dark matter' or 'dark energy', relating to the incredible amount of matter and energy in the Universe (estimated to comprise 97% of it) which is invisible to our methods of detection, but which we *know* is there. Einstein said that to deny ether was to deny the fundamental mechanics of the Universe. While modern science happily abandoned the theory after one faulty and poorly conducted experiment, it has re-emerged various times in physics as a similar concept under the guise of several different names (i.e. 'zero-point' energy) or under a modified theory, such as dark matter and dark energy – which are recognized and discovered factual phenomena, but as yet have not been developed into an encompassing theoretical model of behavior *that will integrate easily into the (seriously flawed) standard model of physics.* Many scientists, with many sound theories, have tried to go up against the seriously flawed standard model of physics, with no success as of yet. It is nearly impossible to change, and is the reason that ether was originally so quickly and adamantly abandoned in the first place. However, now that computer models and detection methods that have confirmed the existence and abundance of what is now called 'dark matter' and 'dark energy' within the Universe, there are many minds scrambling to integrate its presence into their pre-existing models. Whether discussed as ether, dark matter, or dark energy, the fundamental concept remains the same – a mysterious unseen force and apparent source of manifested light, matter, and energy, a cosmic sea in which everything persists. Even the language used to discuss such a concept involves the use of water words, i.e. the sea of energy, ocean of energy, depths of the Universe, etc.

While ether, dark matter, and dark energy are most certainly *not* 'water', the ancient texts clearly display a recognized connection between the ethers of the Universe and its water-like properties – not properties in the sense of water as a physical, chemical substance, but properties in the sense of its responsiveness, memory storage capacities, its ability to structure, and its fluidity and non-static nature. The ancient recognition of this relationship is remarkable, and 'Water' representing the Ether has its place in the beginning or center of every creation story, and as the holiest of holy substances. Every tradition has its own perspective, relations, and retelling of the story "In the beginning…" Yet for all variances in tradition – and some are incredibly large – we encounter a great similarity of description: In the beginning, we have a pervasive notion of the Spirit of God (whether the sun god in Egyptian mythology or the Judeo-Christian God), residing in the waters of the primeval ocean (ether), and the elements of Creation (light, cosmos, earth, matter, etc.) emerging from the primordial sea (ether). These references to 'water' are not intended to describe the physical form of water, which is described later on in most sacred texts as one of the primary substances and elements of Creation and is distinctly different from the 'waters' first mentioned at the *beginning* of the Creation story. No, these first 'waters' are understood to describe the *'ethers'* or *'aethers',* the pervasive sea of energy throughout the Universe. And so it is said that we are as the fish – who know not the water for the sea.

*The earth was without form, and void; and darkness was on the face of the deep. And the Spirit of God was hovering over the face of the waters.*
~BIBLE, OLD TESTAMENT: GENESIS 1:2

This line of Biblical scripture, expressing the existence of water, comes *before* God creates Light, and depicts an entire Universe of "Water" (again water the concept, rather than water the substance). Here the word *'earth'* does not mean our planet Earth, as this had yet to be created. It did not mean oceans or seas, as these were also manifested later. No, this was before the acts of Creation, pre-'big-bang', and the Earth referenced relates to our physical matter, or the physical Universe, which was *without form and void,* and the 'Waters' were the ethers, the dark matter, or the primordial ocean, where *darkness was on the face of the deep.* This early scene in Genesis is one of the most repeated themes throughout the world's many spiritual and religious texts, all expressing the ethers of the Universe:

*In the beginning were Darkness, Chaos, and Water.*
~ST. EPIPHANIUS, PANARION HAER. 25, 5

*In the beginning there was only the Creator. From him the*

*'water' was formed; from the water heated, the 'foam' was formed.*
~RIG VEDA, HYMN OF CREATION ( I. 2.1 )

*There was not the non-existent nor the existent then. A Darkness was in the beginning hidden by darkness. This all was water.*
~ VEDIC CREATION

*First the gods, and subsequently all beings, arose from the fusion of salt water (Tiamat) and sweet water (Apsu).*
~ASSYRO-BABYLONIAN CREATION

*(In the beginning) ...Apsu (sweet water), the first one, their begetter, And maker Tiamat (salt water), who bore them all, Had mixed their waters together... When yet no gods were manifest, Nor names pronounced, nor destinies decreed, Then gods were born within them.*
~MESOPOTAMIAN BABYLONIAN CREATION

*In the Beginning, the sun-god Atum (Amen-Re) resided in Nun, the primordial ocean.*
~EGYPTIAN HELIOPOLITAN CREATION

*In the beginning there is nothingness. Gradually this space filled with water...*
~NORSE CREATION, ORIGINATING FROM NORTHERN EUROPEAN, GERMANIC, SCANDINAVIAN, AND BALTIC TRIBES

*At the beginning of time, Narayana lay floating on the primeval waters. After many ages, Narayana began to create the Universe...*
~EARLY HINDU CREATION

*The first being, named Mbombo, presided over a dark and watery world.*
~BAKUBA CREATION, AFRICA

*In the beginning, in the dark, there was nothing but water.*
~BUSHONGO CREATION, CENTRAL AFRICA

*Thousands of years ago, there was no land nor sun nor moon nor stars, and the world was only a great sea of water.*
~ANCIENT FILIPINO CREATION

*In the beginning, the gods were situated above a primordial body of water.*
~SIBERIAN ALTAIC, NORTH AMERICAN
AND EASTERN EUROPE CREATION (EARTH-DIVER
NARRATIVE)

*In the beginning there was no earth to live on, only a watery abyss.*
~IROQUOIS CREATION

*In the beginning there was only one water.*
~WYANDOT (HURON) CREATION

*In the beginning, there was just water.*
~CHEROKEE CREATION

*In the beginning, Sophia appears as the first Spirit, moving over the waters. Under her are the four material elements – water, darkness, abyss, and chaos.*
~SYRIAN GNOSTIC CREATION

In Gnosticism, Sophia is defined as the Holy Spirit, the

Great Mother principle. Here we see a clear distinction between the waters of ether and the material element of water.

> *Before Creation, it was only the Braham that was*
> *everywhere. There was no day, night, or sky. First I created the*
> *waters.*
> ~VAYU PURANA 4.74, VEDIC CREATION

In Vedic traditions, Braham is defined as the ultimate reality, the eternal ineffable Supreme Godhead.

> *In the beginning there was darkness,*
> *Utter darkness, darkness upon darkness,*
> *The world then was merely its primordial essence,*
> *its inconsistent ocean, its formless fabric.*
> *Thus what would become of this world was first wrapped*
> *within the*
> *All pervading power of the Eternal One*
> *Before whom our material world is but a trifle*
> *brought into existence*
> *By the omnipotent force of His will alone.*
> ~RIG VEDA, THE HYMN OF CREATION (X.129)

The Hymn of Creation, written in Sanskrit, has been interpreted by Vedic scholars as expressing that during the pre-Creation time of the Universe, there was nothing but the bottomless, uninterrupted, limitless 'water' (ether), its *inconsistent ocean*. The Universe is therefore spoken of as having been originally "water" (ether) without light (dark matter). As it identifies the waters as the first residence of the eternal being, water is said to be the underlying principle or the very foundation of the Universe.

*He, whose destination is the ocean, who purifies the world, is always flowing, such water lives in the middle of the Universe.*
~RIG VEDA (X.29.3)

*In the beginning there was nothing. The universe was enveloped by death alone. He produced mind. He moved about worshipping himself. As he was worshipping himself, water was produced.*
~RIG VEDA, HYMN OF CREATION

*There was neither death nor immortality. There was nothing to distinguish night from day. There was no wind or breath. God alone breathed by his own energy. Other than God there was nothing. In the beginning darkness was swathed in darkness. All was liquid and formless. God was clothed in emptiness.*
~RIG VEDA

*He is the One Who created Heaven and Earth in six days. His Throne rises over the water.*
~QUR'AN

All of these references to water refer to the properties of water as energy, the cosmic principle of Water rather than the physical principle of water. Our Universe is permeated with this property, it underlies all things and is a fact acknowledged by nearly all ancient traditions. The structure of the Universe is a living dynamic responsive crystalline matrix, which provides the medium for the manifestation of consciousness and thus the manifestation of all that surrounds us. It is de-structured by lower forms of consciousness, and more highly structured by higher forms of consciousness and those which support it – i.e. crystals or gems, and the fields radiating from the hearts, minds, and bodies of people in the spirit of Love and connection. It is only because of the energetically polluted space on Earth that we cannot view the original structure, so inundated are we with polluted energetics and the disordered de-structuring of our environment. The acknowledgment of the crystalline matrix of the Universe unifies field theories and explains all phenomena. It will never be quantified or calculated in equations, as the only constant is that it is never constant. Its variables are fluid, ever-changing and non-static, and the synergism of energetic and consciousness interactions continue to increase the dimensionally fractal Field which appears to the observer to expand as its grows in depth and fractality, creating more dimensions as it creates more intricacy of structures for pattern interactions. While it cannot be calculated, it can be understood, and this understanding applied for the betterment of Mankind. It is Source energetic controlling every particle of Life that exists within its Matrix, refracting and reflecting all frequencies of Life in manifestation. Every science is pointing to the intelligence of "The Field." Structured Energetics is its Intelligence.

*...and the mirrors and lenses of space which are the cause of illusion in all moving things.*
~WALTER RUSSELL
THE SECRET OF LIGHT

# RESOURCES

<u>POND AND LAKE RESTORATION/REHABILITATION:</u>

Employ effective, long-term, natural solutions, and work with a dedicated team capable of restoring and rehabilitating virtually any water system. From home ponds to wastewater sites and ocean bays, toxic algae, foul oder, and unusable waterways, we are intent on improving and restoring our waters, and work to provide the restoration needed for any project size. Contact carly@watercodes.com for more information on pond or lake restoration.

<u>WATER TREATMENT SYSTEMS:</u>

Did you know that in addition to holding the key to obtain optimal health and longevity, your water – whether tap, bottled, or basic filtered, is also still likely your greatest source of toxic exposure? Our systemic pollution has made complete and total purification an essential step.

Investing in an effective purification system and remineralization system is the single greatest way to reduce you and your family's toxic exposure to harmful carcinogens, pollutants, micro-plastics, and disinfecting byproducts. Becoming self-sufficient for your drinking water needs is the safest, most healthy, and most sustainable solution. Unfortunately, the overwhelming majority of purifications systems on the market do not perform anywhere near claims. To create a truly quality Water at home, one would follow a three stage process requiring purification, remineralization, and restructuring. Currently, TrueSpring is the only company I know that offers a hospital grade purification system followed by an effective broad spectrum remineralization system. Contact **nevin@truestspring.com** for more information or to acquire one of these effective systems for yourself.

## WATER STRUCTURING SYSTEMS:

Structuring systems are being continually developed and improved. For more information on structuring systems I currently recommend, please feel free to contact me at carly@watercodes.com.

## DIY WATER STRUCTURING SOLUTIONS:

There are a variety of DIY options available for water structuring! Of course, the structure of water is on a spectrum and has varying degrees of structure, and not every system whether purchased or DIY will result in highly structured water. It will, however, undoubtedly have some kind of an effect and is a great place to start with minimal investment. In my experience and research, most (though not all) of the systems available on the market do not create a structure in water that is any better than the DIY solutions described here, or found and created elsewhere – the internet has plenty of suggestions. If you have questions while developing your own DIY system, or for serious structuring systems (non-DIY), contact me at carly@watercodes.com By applying the principles of structured water physics, you can create a beginner's system at home! Some suggested DIY options include:

- Homemade filtration systems using magnetite, shungite, or other crystals and minerals,

- Magnetite Storage Solution: wherein water is stored in a container (preferably glass) overnight while (mostly) submerged in a bucket of magnetite,

- DIY Shower Filtration Systems: by purchasing a shower filter with removable ceramic beads, you can replace these beads with various crystals and minerals for an improved water structure – I suggest eBay for shower filter options,

- DIY Glass Ball water "filter": a homemade water conditioner can be made using simple marbles, and allowing water to pass over the marbles several times, mimicking some market units for a fraction of the cost.

EMF SOLUTIONS:

As a consumer, I have tried multiple devices and products available on the market. I am happy to give you my experience with different technologies before investing yourself. In addition to the technology that I use, my suggestions may vary depending on your needs and objectives. Contact    carly@watercodes.com    for    my suggestions and recommendations.

**RECOMMENDED READING:**

*Life's Matrix: A Biography of Water*
Philip Ball, 2001.

In *Life's Matrix,* Philip Ball writes of water's origins, history, and unique physical character. As a geological agent, water shapes mountains, canyons, and coastlines, and when unleashed in hurricanes and floods its destructive power is awesome. Philip goes just deep enough into chemistry, physics, geology, and environmental science to infuse you with the journey. *Life's Matrix* also examines the grim realities of depletion of natural resources and its effects on the availability of water in the twenty-first century.

*Hidden Nature: The Startling Insights of Viktor Schauberger*
Alick Bartholomew, 2004.

This book describes and explains Schauberger's insights in contemporary, accessible language. His remarkable discoveries — which address issues such as sick water, ailing forests, climate change, and renewable energy — have dramatic implications for how we should work with nature and its resources. Alick was the original publisher bringing Schauberger's works into English. Accessible and relevant, it shows how Schauberger's work can be effectively used in dealing with today's environmental challenges.

**Primary Perception: Biocommunication with Plants, Living Foods, and Human Cells**
Cleve Backster, 2003.

Cleve Backster is a polygraph expert who, for over 54 years, has maintained his status in the field of "Psychophysiology" [polygraph] and runs the Backster School of Lie Detection in San Diego, California. The book covers 36 years in which he has made numerous discoveries in bio-communication. This is the only book about his work by Cleve Backster himself.

**Tuning into Nature**
Philip Callahan, 2001.

Phil Callahan reveals the miraculous communication systems present in nature and provides a fascinating and fantastic account of the complexity of nature and her communication systems.

**Paramagnetism: Rediscovering Nature's Secret Force of Growth**
Philip Callahan, 1995

Callahan shares his depth of knowledge and research into the low-frequency forces in nature and the effects of the paramagnetic force on soils, plants, and people.

*Living Energies: An Exposition of Concepts Related to the Theories of Viktor Schauberger*
Callum Coats, 2001.

This popular, brilliant book is the definitive textbook on the works and the modern applications of forester, scientist and pioneering inventor Viktor Schauberger. A must-read if you want to understand, research, and apply naturalist technologies. Comprehensively analyzes natural implosion and explosion, and the regenerative and degenerative processes.

*Spiritual Nutritions: Six Foundations for Spiritual Life*
Gabriel Cousens, 2005.

With years of clinical experience and research, Dr Cousens discusses energy, diet, meditation, and kundalini in thorough and technical detail in an amazing book full of information. Through supported lessons, Cousens teaches us that diet and fasting has an effect on our energy levels and spiritual development, and outlines his conclusions on how to build a successful and spiritually supportive diet and lifestyle.

*Messages from Water – Vol. 1, Vol. 2, Vol. 3*
Masaru Emoto, 1999+.

This series of books illustrates experiments with frozen water crystals formed from a wide variety of water sources, and illustrates photographic research demonstrating the visual effects of the quality of energy in water. Clean pure water from natural and unpolluted sources makes brilliant and sparkling snowflake patterns, rich in color and luminosity. By contrast, polluted waters show flat and dull patterns lacking in structure or color. Bilingual editions, Japanese and English, with color photos on nearly every page.

### *The Hidden Messages in Water*
Masaru Emoto, 2007.

An introduction to Emoto's study of water and the power of words and sounds to affect water molecules. Filled with illustrations and detailed accounts of experiments that inspire wonder.

### *Vibrational Medicine*
Richard Gerber, 2001.

The #1 handbook of subtle energy sciences, *Vibrational Medicine* is a comprehensive guide to energetic healing and the textbook of choice for an introduction to the study of alternative medicine. Dr. Gerber provides an encyclopedic treatment and reference material of energetic healing, covering a variety of topics within the field. He explains current theories about how various therapies work and offers new insights into the physical and spiritual perspectives of health and disease.

### *Cymatics: A Study of Wave Phenomenon*
Hans Jenny, 2001.

Documenting 14 years of meticulous experiments using audible sound to display flowing forms. Over 350 stunning photographs reflect patterns found throughout nature, inspiring deep recognition of the power of sound and vibration.

### Sound Water Images: The Creative Music of the Universe
Alexander Lauterwasser, 2007.

In this collection of awe-inspiring images, photographer and researcher Alexander Lauterwasser sheds new light on the famous sand figures of Ernst Chladni, which fascinated Napoleon at the turn of the 19th Century, as well as Dr. Hans Jenny's Cymatic sound forms of the 1950's and 60's, to create a new scientific art form for the modern day.

### The Holy Order of Water: Healing the Earth's Waters and Ourselves
William Marks, 2001.

Healing Earth's Waters and Ourselves discusses a kaleidoscopic variety of subjects including water and the human body, vortex energy, cosmic rain, the use of water in spiritual practices, healing with water, and much more.

### Deep: Freediving, Renegade Science, and What the Ocean Tells Us About Ourselves
James Nestor, 2015.

Deep delves into mysterious ocean phenomena, and discusses how amazing abilities of ocean creatures are reflected in our own remarkable and often hidden potential, and the profound bodily changes humans undergo when underwater.

*Blue Mind: The Surprising Science That Shows How Being Near, In, On, or Under Water Can Make You Happier, Healthier, More Connected, and Better at What You Do*
Wallace J. Nichols, 2015.

In *Blue Mind*, Wallace J. Nichols revolutionizes how we think about being near water, and uses neuroscience and psychology, as well as personal stories from leading scientists, top athletes, gifted artists, and others, to reveal the remarkable benefits of being in, on, under, or simply near water. *Blue Mind* illustrates how proximity to water can improve performance, increase calm, diminish anxiety, and increase professional success.

*The Fourth Phase of Water: Beyond Solid, Liquid, and Vapor*
Gerald Pollack, 2013.

Professor Gerald Pollack provides a fantastic journey through water, and in simple ways helps the reader understand how changes in water's structure underlie most energetic transitions of form and motion on earth. Amazing material with revolutionary insights, Pollack provides the easy to understand explanation of water as an aqueous gel that holds and conducts electricity.

*The Healing Energies of Water*
Charlie Ryrie, 1999.

Tracing the development of human relationships with water. From primitive healing cults to the most recent scientific studies, this thoughtful volume explores water's role in our spirituality, folklore and myth.

*Water Crystals: Making the Quality of Water Visible*
Andreas Schulz, 2005.

The quality of our water—especially drinking water—is becoming an increasingly important issue. Andreas Schulz uses a photographic process to make the quality of various kinds of water instantly visible to the non-specialist. Using water samples from many parts of the world, this remarkable and beautiful book provides a unique insight into the world of water.

*Sensitive Chaos*
Theodor Schwenk, 2001.

"Water is more than a mere flow of energy or a useful means of transport." Lavishly illustrated, Sensitive Chaos shows the unifying forces which underlie all living things. The book illuminates phenomena from birds' flight to movements of fish, to air patterns in musical instruments. It observes the formation of internal organs; mountain ranges and river deltas; sand patterns on the beach and even the human embryo.

*Water, the Element of Life*
Theodor Schwenk, 2000.

The living movement of water makes life on earth possible. Based on Rudolf Steiner's Anthroposophy and their own numerous experiments, Theodore and Wolfram Schwenk show that the earth is a living organism and that water is its sense organ. Water perceives vital cosmic influences and forces and transforms these into earthly life.

*Energizing Water: Flowform Technology and the Power of Nature*
John Wilkes, et al, 2010.

Rhythms and flow have a positive effect on the capacity of water to support life. *Energizing Water* discusses the background story of the research and application of the flowform method today, a creative technology using nature's methods to produce results.

ABOUT THE AUTHOR

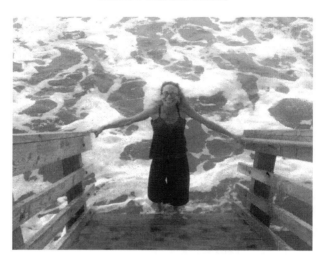

Carly Nuday has been studying water, bio-water, health, consciousness, and energy sciences her entire life. In 2011 she co-patented a technology used in bio-water restructuring, and was senior researcher and Director of Water, Inc., a non-profit dedicated to the education, advancement, and development of water science. Dedicated to restoring Water both inside and outside the body, today Carly works with both bio-water technologies as well as the most effective, long-term, and natural solutions for pond and lake restorations and rehabilitations.

carly@watercodes.com

Made in the USA
Las Vegas, NV
05 November 2022